UNDERSTANDING REIKI

FROM SELF-CARE TO ENERGY MEDICINE

Chyna Honey

ISBN: 978-1-4834-1937-4 (sc)
ISBN: 978-1-4834-1936-7 (e)

Library of Congress Control Number: 2014917873

Lulu Publishing Services rev. date: 10/14/2014

DEDICATION

To the curious who picked this book up, but even more,
to the courageous who read it through to the end.

Thank You

To my many teachers: the Reiki Master Teachers of my lineage, my Energy Medicine Instructors, and to the clients that taught me more through their words, energy and experience than any book could. May this book be a worthy reflection of the information you have shared, and teachings you have given.

A few special thank yous

To my friend, teacher and husband, Jim Honey. Thank you Jim for your support, ideas, sounding board impersonations, cups of warm tea, and for the endless number of puns, funny faces and light hearted jokes that made writing a book, one of the hardest things I've ever done, something I've thoroughly enjoyed and grown from.

To my friends Tiffany & Reggie Hunter, who helped in reading the drafts and in sharing their many reactions to what is written here, all while offering words & actions of endless encouragement.

And a special and additional thank you to Tiffany Hunter, who upon the book's completion, agreed to be my editing partner, which meant spending hours drinking tea while discussing Reiki and the wonders of correct punctuation. With a serene sense of humor and a commitment to see this book in the world, she gave her time and energy to support it and me. In our time together editing and discussing, and at the bottom of a deep and seemingly endless cup of tea, we found what we did not think was possible, a new love for the use and teaching of Reiki.

Reiki is the name given to a particular natural, healing vibration that is of great benefit to humans.

Reiki is also the name of a formalized healing practice that uses this particular vibration to aid humans, in living with greater ease, and enjoy better quality of life.

Reiki is one of many natural healing vibrations that co-exist within our shared environment and has a specific purpose.

This book explains in great detail what Reiki is, what it isn't and why Reiki is essential to our daily self-care.

Contents

PURPOSE

The purpose of this book is to provide information on what Reiki is, its role as an essential self-care practice, and how it can benefit others as a form of Energy Medicine. It provides insights and points of discussion for Reiki Masters and Master Teachers to expand their understanding of the healing system they have dedicated themselves to learning, while also using its content to reconsider how Reiki is taught to students today.

These are key considerations for the reader at any level of Reiki understanding, and if what I have written so far intrigues you, I encourage you to read on. If however, you are seeking information on Reiki as a means to use it as a spiritual or meditative practice, then not only is this book not for you, but Reiki itself is not for you, because Reiki is neither a spiritual or meditative practice.

Reiki is a healing vibration of great use and benefit to humans. Its practice does not require a meditative state or a desire for spiritual awakening, and its benefits go beyond what a meditative state alone provides. This is not to say that meditation, as a practice does not have its merits; it certainly does. This is simply not the book that discusses those benefits, or limits its understanding of Reiki to meditation or spiritual endeavors.

With that said, the confusion that it does these things is understandable when you consider that the benefits inherent in a consistent practice of Reiki may make the journey of a spiritual path easier and provide greater depth to a meditative practice. The result of this confusion, however, is that there are many books written about Reiki that speak of it from this perspective, and in so doing, make a promise that Reiki can provide a path to enlightenment or a way to meditate and bring in a higher power, that Reiki is not meant to keep. Furthermore, when Reiki is perceived to have failed in keeping that promise, one of two things happen; either the person trying feels they have failed Reiki, or that Reiki has failed them. The result is commonly the abandonment of its use, which will bring about a host of other problems, felt, but not understood.

It is in this spirit then, that this book embarks on a journey to explain in a clear and concise manner what Reiki is and what it isn't. It does this by giving you specifics with which to examine Reiki from a new vantage point. In doing so, it provides a learning and understanding that encourages and inspires more people on the planet to begin using this incredibly pure and natural healing vibration as a means to improve health and provide a better quality of life.

How to Best Use This Book

What makes this book different is its presentation of Reiki as a form of Energy Medicine. By placing it back into the realm from which it always belonged, this book provides clear information on how and why a consistent practice of Reiki supports the health and well-being of humans. To do this means to speak and to consider Reiki in a new way, which neither relies on scientific explanations, nor is dependent on the belief that Reiki is the work of a higher, unexplainable power, that brings humans in contact with their higher selves to receive healing.

At times, it will step out of the Reiki conversation to provide additional information that will help the reader better understand Reiki in this greater context. This may on occasion leave you feeling that the information provided is a bit intense or requires contemplation. My friends and I jokingly call this the "getting up to make a cup of tea effect", which describes the moment when you have read something that challenges you in a new way and you need to take a moment to allow it to soak in. If this is your experience, I encourage you to make and enjoy a cup of tea, or do whatever simple activity you enjoy to help you relax. Doing this will give you time to contemplate and integrate the information being shared. If you do, you give yourself the opportunity to take the information provided and use it to gain a deeper understanding of Reiki and possibly yourself.

While this is certainly a book that can be read once, and relegated to the bookshelf, doing so limits the reader's opportunity to gain a greater and deeper understanding of Reiki. For understanding and knowledge is acquired over time as a part of practice. As the individual changes and evolves throughout the span of his or her life, information is perceived through that experience, and knowledge gained naturally evolves. So then, this book is written to provide you with road signs and a map with options of travel, as you begin and continue on your journey of Reiki.

While this book is filled with many words, it also contains levels of energy information that can only be received at the reader's current level of understanding. As your practice deepens and evolves, so will what you can get from this book. There are opportunities available and offered at any level of interest the reader has, from the curious, to the keenly adept.

What is certain is that this book will challenge what the reader knows about the level of self-care required for all humans to live and enjoy life with greater ease. This is exciting, because unlike so many of the challenges humans are faced with, it comes with answers and information that empowers the individual to care for themselves and the people they care about in a new way.

May you enjoy all that follows…

ONE

BREAKING AWAY

These pages provide a breaking away from how Reiki is spoken, written about and taught in the current age. It contains information in a context not shared before, and in this way significantly diverges from how Reiki is thought about today.

It is with great reverence, love and care for Reiki and its teaching that I share what I do here. While I understand that some of what is shared may be unpopular, it is written as a means to shift focus back to feeling Reiki and allowing the vibration and its teachings to inform the person using it. This is a challenge, because while the concept itself is easy enough to understand, our western culture has an established way of teaching that focuses on facts to engage the mind, and places greater value on the strength of our mental processes than the natural innate learning abilities of our body. Furthermore, it tends to focus on content, more so than on the quality, and care of instruction.

So our journey begins by providing reminders that what is lost when the student is encouraged to focus on achievement by acquiring facts, is the richness found in the experience of learning.

1

BALANCING ORAL TRADITION WITH WRITTEN TEXT

Reiki was originally taught as an oral tradition and kept simple for people at all levels across the social, economic and educational spectrum to use and understand. This made the information immediately and freely accessible to any member of the human race able to hear the information. This bypassed class, gender, economic or any other form of classification used to discriminate or define value to a human being. The value of this cannot be underestimated.

Learning through an oral tradition is enhanced through the quality of the relationship and trust established between the teacher and student. Both have long valued this tradition for enabling the teacher to teach at a pace the student can learn from, thereby creating a dialogue that empowers the student to both process and exercise the information as its being taught. It provides flexibility that makes it possible for a teacher to teach multiple students simultaneously, while making the level of information provided unique to each student.

However, the key problem inherent in the oral tradition is that it is difficult to keep the information pure. This is because all information heard and received is subject to interpretation. In the United States kids illustrate this in a game called Telephone in which a group of people sit in a circle. It then starts by one person whispering something into the ear of the next person, and then that person whispering the information they heard to the person next to them, and so on, until the information is whispered into the ear of the last remaining person yet to hear it. Finally, the person who received the information last shares aloud what they heard with the group. The final message, now being compared to the original message, is commonly received with laughter and wonder as each member of the game marvels at how the simple message at the start has changed into a very different message by the end. This game has also been called Chinese Whispers and by other names in different cultures. What is of interest, is that every culture has their own version of this game, and has used it as a tool to illustrate how difficult it is, even among a small group, to maintain the integrity of information passed orally.

In a growing effort to maintain the integrity of information given, and to minimize the effects of our human tendency towards exaggeration or distortion, people began writing things down. While this practice was well intended, it proved prone to the same problems; especially as the audience grew and the information was passed on to new and different cultures.

The result today is that you will find much well intentioned, albeit misinformed information, about Reiki in bookstores, online and in practice. While most of it was created to provide information and answer questions about the practice, it has left students feeling insecure about what they have received. This is because while they have received a lot of information, they are not given what they need most, the confidence in practice that comes when understanding of a subject is realized.

This causes different reactions in people. Because humans naturally devalue what they don't understand, some will abandon the practice over time because they can't explain it to themselves or to the people they care about. Others will try to make it into something new, something they can understand, explain and teach to others, and in essence, make it their own.

In this way, and in most cases, complications and misinformation is spread by well meaning Reiki Master Teachers doing what they can to try to validate a pure and ancient practice. The problem is, as with most things human, that understanding is sought by complicating something, instead of studying its simplicity and purity.

What is required then, is to take Reiki back, in practice and in instruction, from the written amalgamation of descriptions and techniques, into the simplicity and purity originally taught as an oral tradition. While no book can achieve such a task or in any way take the place of a true oral tradition, this book is written to reclaim the information as a means to restore and instill an understanding of Reiki that in effect draws people towards its practice.

VALUE OF THE MASTER TEACHER/STUDENT RELATIONSHIP

In the West, the value of the Master Teacher/Student relationship has gone the same way of Oral Traditions, in that it has been diminished and partially replaced. Despite the fact that our Western culture places greater value on quantity of content than it does quality of instruction, what is remembered and valued by most students, is the teachers they met and the influence the teacher(s) had on their learning experience. It is these relationships then, for either positive or negative reasons, which leave a greater impression on the student and are so remembered with greater clarity than the details of the instruction once received.

We live in an age where online courses are commonplace. This shift is not new or a reflection of technological advancements, but rather cultural, and is merely an extension of the older mail-order courses offered in the 1950's. While there is no argument that there are benefits to this form of instruction, it is more of a drive-thru method of learning and it comes at great cost to the aspiring student, eager to learn and to grow within a certain course of study.

Reiki is more than a course of study. By missing or having lost that information it becomes ever easier to value the consumption of facts and information over the need to understand and use through practice.

This book is written in support of, and in reverence to, the Master Teacher/Student relationship. It holds that no book, website, DVD set or online seminar can or should attempt to usurp the value and depth of knowledge that can be attained through this direct form of tutelage. This book, then, strives to stay away from details generally provided as part of the instruction given in a Reiki attunement. Instead, it is written to support and add value to that relationship by providing information not readily available or shared, while also striving to open new points of discussion for consideration of how Reiki is currently taught. Its emphasis throughout is on the value of pairing direct experience with clear instruction. This is best attained by working with a Master Teacher that is committed to helping you further your personal practice in their effort to progress and promote the practice of Reiki. Generally speaking this is done through regular and consistent practice that, accompanied by clear instruction, is further supported by answering questions as they arise. In this way, the Master

Teacher empowers and allows the rate at which the student can learn to dictate the stream of when new and additional information and training can be offered.

PROGRESSING REIKI INSTRUCTION

The next three points will help to illustrate how students have been brought to focus on things related to Reiki, but are not Reiki. Instead they offer information that can inadvertently get in the way of the student's learning. Through this examination, the opportunity to return to learning through personal experience is presented. While its content may provoke some, put off by its break with traditional teaching formats, it is likely to provide relief to others who learn best through a combination of feeling, discussing and doing. For Reiki Masters and Master Teachers this is an opportunity to progress the teachings by bringing it back to its roots.

No History Lesson Here

In this book I will not discuss the history of Reiki or the man considered its founder, Master Mikao Usui. It is because I have great reverence for Master Usui that I avoid going into explanations about him and the journey that is credited to him for bringing an awareness of Reiki into the world of human consciousness.

While Master Usui gave Reiki its name and a focused structure that engenders learning and understanding, I feel that he would want students of Reiki to focus their attention and experience on using Reiki, rather than focusing on his personal qualities, or on what led him to find Reiki, and spend the remainder of his lifetime teaching others how to use and benefit from it. For it is in the vibration itself, not the man or the collection of Reiki Master Teachers, both men and women who followed him, that the purity of Reiki and the knowledge within can be found.

NOT FROM JAPAN

Reiki has long been called and considered a Japanese healing system. This is misleading because most do not effectively differentiate between the vibration and the formalized healing system that was developed as a means to share its benefits through use.

Reiki is a natural, healing vibration for humans, and so holds no cultural identity or passport. It is a vibration that benefits the human energy system, and by identifying it with a culture and a nationality, it potentially quarantines its use to people that share that affiliation or have interest in the culture and nationality highlighted and credited as its creator.

The vibration was re-discovered, named, formalized and then shared by a man, who was born in Japan. Once he understood the vibration he formalized a system around it and dedicated the remainder of his life to teaching others how to use it to improve health and quality of life. Master Usui gave us a name for the vibration and a formalized system designed to help others use and establish value for the vibration. Giving the vibration a cultural identity was not an intention of Master Usui, it is simply a consequence of his personal country of origin. Identifying it culturally or in any other way adds no value, and in fact can inadvertently cause division by establishing a false sense of ownership.

Imagine for a moment if eating food was given a cultural identity. In reality, it can't. Utensils used to facilitate eating were designed by different cultures and those societies then taught a system that facilitated eating, but understanding how to use those tools, may make eating easier and certainly cleaner it does little to nourish to body, and that after all is the point.

To deeply understand Reiki, all one needs to do is to use and feel the vibration. Reading history or studying mythologies will not inform you of the purity and benefits received through its use. It will however, provide a framework for the mind, which is the reason they are used for instruction. The benefit to this, is it that the framework of this system may help you to better connect to and use the vibration. The limitation of this however is if the student places more value on the framework of the system than on the vibration itself. For it is the vibration that heals, not the mind's interpretation of the vibration or the history of its formalized system, or knowing the names of the Reiki Master Teachers that preceded you as the student. By getting back to the true intention of Master Usui, which was getting people to use the vibration on a regular and consistent basis, we re-introduce the vibration to the whole of the species it is intended to heal. To be successful we need to avoid identifying it by subsets within the human species.

No Pictures Of Positions And No Symbols

This book will not include images of people receiving Reiki and the various positions on the body where Reiki is delivered as part of a Reiki session, because this is information you will receive, or have received, during the attunement process with your Master Teacher. This book will also not include any Reiki symbols.

The passing of images and information on Reiki symbols is a sacred part of the Reiki Level II and Master attunement levels. It is a personal gift to allow yourself not to see or encounter a symbol until you are ready to use it. That readiness comes as part of your initiation into these higher attunement levels. Waiting until such initiation takes place, will provide you, and imbue the process you will go through with greater opportunity for knowledge and power.

Besides, until you start that initiation process, a process that cannot be rushed and so should not be; you are simply not ready for the information and as such it will have no value to you. This is often the problem with books and widely available written material. It provides information in a general context without consideration of meeting a student at the level of teaching they are able to receive at any one time. This is why written information should support, but not usurp, oral instruction, or attempt to take the place of the Master Teacher/ Student relationship.

For the overly eager Reiki student, the result of rushing to attain new information, or giving into curiosity, will in the end, dilute it. When this happens, the student loses out on an opportunity for learning that paces instruction with experience. For the teacher eager to impress others with their knowledge and insights, you risk robbing the student of a sacred coming of age in Reiki. It is for this reason that it is unfair and unwise for a Reiki Master Teacher to be cavalier with the symbols or to place them in a book for the general public to see.

If you are a student who has yet to see a symbol, I encourage waiting and doing what you can to avoid them if they come into view. Give yourself the gift of experiencing them when you are ready for your Reiki Level II or Master level attunements. Then, you will not only receive the image, but the vibrational information contained within them, which goes far beyond what the images alone and general descriptions provide.

Two

Introducing & Explaining Reiki

Knowledge on any subject is achieved through the combination of two things: by satisfying the mind's need for information and the body's need for direct experience. Memorizing facts or genealogies of lineages, or another person's interpretation of ancient texts, will appease the mind's need for information, but it will not bring you closer to feeling and knowing Reiki. To know for yourself what Reiki is and isn't, you will need to trust yourself and balance the reading you do and the instruction you receive from your Reiki Master Teacher, with your direct experience. In doing so, the student takes responsibility for his or her exploration and learning. While the responsibility of any teacher is to show the student the way to greater knowledge, the responsibility of every student is to use the information and direction provided by pairing it with practice, also referred to here as direct experience. When this is done, the student will then know if what is shared is true and correct, if it is not, or if something has changed. It is in this knowing that instruction and acquisition of information is transformed into knowledge.

Many can attest to the experience of reading or hearing something and knowing without reservation that the information is true. It is a quiet but unmistakable knowing. This is the feeling you are after for it is the seat of your inner wisdom, which is pliable and always changing, yet constant and unyielding in its pursuit to know through direct experience.

In this pursuit, if you have been attuned to Reiki at any level, consider reading the remainder of this chapter, as well as other parts of this book, with your cupped Reiki hand[1] placed somewhere comfortable on your body. By doing so you are giving yourself the opportunity to learn while boosting its content with the experience of receiving Reiki as you read.

EXPLAINING REIKI TO ANOTHER

When I am explaining what Reiki is, I often do so by asking the person I am about to explain it to, to extend his or her hand out to me, palm up, and allow me to show them. I do this by placing my hand over their hand in the cupped Reiki hand position. This starts the flow of Reiki from my hand into their hand. I will then ask the person to let me know when they feel something. Once they do, I begin my explanation.

In my experience, most people feel the Reiki vibration within about 5-15 seconds. They may not be sure what they are feeling, but they feel something. Some will describe this new sensation as heat, while others may describe it as a buzzing, and still others will say they're not sure how to describe what they feel, but they know they feel something. It is at this

---

[1] The cupped Reiki hand position is described and discussed in greater detail in Chapter 5.

moment that the person has acknowledged to their mind that their body is feeling the natural healing vibration of Reiki. The feeling, although new to the mind, has been known by the body since its birth and is as natural to it as water. It is natural, soothing and relaxing to the human body, even as it is experienced as something unknown and new by the mind. For this reason, I have never seen a person pull their hand away until I have pulled back, stopping the flow of Reiki into their hand.

When the person has accepted and is enjoying this new sensation, I begin my explanation. I do this because it enables the person to learn in two ways; through the direct experience of receiving Reiki, and through my words that describe what the vibration they are beginning to feel is, and what it is doing. This kind of learning satisfies the mind's need for information, and the body's need for experience.

What is Reiki

In simple terms, Reiki is a pure, natural, human energy vibration that provides healing to the physical and auric layers of the human body.

Reiki helps to alleviate physical pain, promotes the biologically necessary relaxation instinct, which in turn, boosts the natural healing abilities of humans. It does this by strengthening and balancing our base connection to the natural environment (earth element) with our ability to astral project to higher planes of consciousness (air element). The balance of these elements, and others, are essential for a healthy, well-balanced human being.

This brief explanation can be quite dense. This is true both for people experiencing Reiki for the first time, and for people that have been practicing it for years. It is an explanation that is simple in its format but profound in its depth. For this reason, it can be visited and revisited many times over and if you are a student of Reiki (at any level) you are encouraged to do so. For in reality, it is a springboard from which more detailed information can come through practice.

A Brief Word About Vibration

Feeling the vibration of Reiki is not unlike placing your hand on your voice box and feeling the vibration that accompanies the sound your voice makes on your fingertips. While your ears listen to the sound, your fingertips feel the vocal vibration. So then, is the voice the sound you hear or the reverberation you feel to the touch? It is both and it is more. For vibration is experienced both through the gross and the subtle[2] senses. Furthermore, there are aspects of vibration that although not perceived by human experience, affect it. Vibration, like all things described, exists on a spectrum that goes from gross to subtle. In the greater world of vibration, sound is of a grosser nature than Reiki. However, both affect human experience.

It has been long known and accepted that sound, particularly experienced through music, affects human

[2] I use the energy definitions of words "gross" and "subtle" throughout the book. Gross refers to what is obvious and immediately perceived through the five senses and subtle refers to what is, but is not obvious or immediately perceivable through the five senses.

emotions. Now science is looking into how infrasound, that is sound waves with frequencies so low that they fall below the lower limit of what is audible to the human eardrum, affect humans. There is growing evidence that suggests it does in many ways, ranging from emotional responses to affecting physical discomfort and developing ailments. What this points to is that more is known than accepted and discussed about how vibrations, even those not experienced through our gross senses, can and do affect us.

It is said, and rightfully so, that everything is vibration. To take that further, vibration is energy and energy is everything.

Why Reiki is Necessary

If you are reading this book, it has likely come to you because on some level you understand that the human form requires more care than the physical or chemical components that can be observed by the scientific community. And you are right! Throughout the course of the day, the human body comes in contact and is affected by a variety of energies/vibrations that co-exist with us on the planet. Most of these energies are forces unseen and of a nature not easily perceived by the mind and body. However, perceived or not, these energies/vibrations affect us and have for time immemorial. In short, Reiki is the energetic remedy to recover from the effects these energies have on our form.

INFORMATION LOST

The energy information that provided the understanding of the care required to sustain and optimize the health of humans was lost, hidden and destroyed over and throughout the course of human history. This resulted in humans losing ancient knowledge and therapies of self-care.

The general consensus among differing schools of thought states that the human body is composed of 60% water, which helps to underscore the importance of maintaining a hydration level that promotes optimal health and functioning. Now imagine for a moment if the benefits of water usage would have been lost in this way? I realize this is a gross example (water being of a physical nature), and extreme by comparison, but I use it to make the point that much of what has been lost is the understanding of how the human body is affected through the use or absence of use of Reiki.

The human body is all energy in different forms and consists of both gross and subtle anatomy. While as a species we have a good understanding of what our gross anatomy does, and have a good idea of how to care for it through proper diet, exercise, drinking plenty of clean water, and being on a regular sleep cycle, we have very little information about what our subtle anatomy does and even less on how we should care for it. While Reiki can do little to inform us on the former, it does a great deal on helping us with the latter.

In addition to caring for the physical body, all human beings require energy vibrations that help to restore health and balance while replenishing our energy system. By its nature, and through the solidity of its system, Reiki is our first line of defense and remedy to recover from the energetic toll these unseen energies and forces have on us.

REIKI'S ROLE IN OUR GENERAL HEALTH

The Reiki vibration is solid and robust by nature. What this means is that it is a consistent energy vibration that is closed to all kinds of influence and manipulation[3]. For this reason, all humans can be attuned to become a channel for Reiki and learn its information through experience and instruction. In fact, it could be argued that it is the personal responsibility of all humans to become attuned to and use the Reiki vibration in consistent and regular practice, for without it; a depth of self-care cannot be realized.

In terms of our general health, Reiki is a self-care, home remedy, and an advanced care practice. This covers the spectrum of general care for a human being, which includes, self-care rituals performed daily or on a regular basis, home remedies provided to friends and family that may or may not be able to provide their own self-care, as well as advanced care treatments, received by a professional and made on demand or as needed.

Becoming attuned and using Reiki will provide you with a much-needed level of self-care that is being missed. To further optimize your self-care practice, it is best accompanied by the advanced care of scheduling periodic "check-ups" by scheduling a 60-minute Reiki session with a Reiki professional. In this way, the self-care practice of Reiki can be compared to the daily practice of brushing and flossing one's teeth. While

---

[3] This is discussed in greater detail in the next chapter.

the advanced care can be compared to benefits received by regularly seeing your Dental Hygienist. The Dental Hygienist, like a Reiki Professional, can help improve and boost the benefits achieved through regular and consistent practice. This is generally achieved by the professionals' ability to go deeper, possibly catching and bringing your attention to blind spots, and in helping to provide new and in-depth information that can help you do a better job in your self-care regime. However, for those wary of dental comparisons, I will say that unlike the trip the Dental Hygienist, receiving Reiki from a Reiki professional is a wonderfully relaxing and enjoyable experience that can end with a deepening of previously received instruction and a new appreciation of practice and self-care.

There are limits, however, to the level of advanced care that can be expected from Reiki, and that Reiki provides. This is discussed in varying detail in the next two chapters.

THREE

UNDERSTANDING REIKI'S PLACE IN ENERGY MEDICINE

Energy Medicine seeks to understand human health, and its experience, in terms of energy. This provides a broader perspective by offering a wider body of knowledge that includes the following: humans are made up of subtle and gross energies; humans are affected by subtle and gross energies that exist within a shared environment; natural, healing energy vibrations exist that can and do provide relief, remedy and balance where health and well-being have become compromised; and all healing traditions (Western, Eastern, Indigenous, etc.) offer valuable information and serve a purpose, but are limited *if* treatment is provided solely to parts of an individual, without consideration of the whole. It is in the last point and truth that the birth of the "holistic" approach has emerged in healthcare today, and its awareness and popularity is growing within both self-care and advanced-care regimes.

The primary practice of Energy Medicine is to use natural, healing vibrations that provide remedy and restore balance to the bodies[4] that make up the human form. Successful practice requires sufficient knowledge and understanding of: gross and subtle human anatomy, and what affects its balance and health; a thorough understanding and training in the use of many natural, energy vibrations; and the personal balance required to heal others with indifference.

Reiki is one of many natural, energy vibrations that restore balance and bring about remedy. In this regard, Reiki is one of many tools that can be used in an Energy Medicine practice. Energy Medicine practitioners, like Reiki students, Masters and Master Teachers, understand that the human body is affected by the many energies/vibrations co-existing within our shared environment, and that these energies affect us in unseen and degenerative ways. Both Energy Medicine and Reiki principles accept and seek to understand the impact these energies have on us, and the toll these energies take on our bodies as a means to provide remedy.

<u>REIKI'S RETURN TO ENERGY MEDICINE</u>

Bringing the discussion of Reiki back into an Energy Medicine context provides a framework that makes Reiki easier to understand and explore. It's a framework that allows us to see it for what it is, what it isn't, what it does, and what it does not do. For understanding Reiki in this way brings us closer to understanding the depth and breadth of the vibration, and why we need to include it as part of our daily self-care regime.

---

[4] A discussion on the bodies that make up the human form is found later in the chapter. In the meantime, consider them parts that make up our form that are inter-related and influence one another.

Reiki is a natural, energy vibration that restores balance and repairs damage in two of the five bodies that make up the human form. While it works directly on only two of the bodies, it works with, and in harmony with, all. This means that Reiki has no contraindications or side effects. It also means that Reiki is as natural to the human energy system as water is to the human body. For this reason, Reiki is a necessary practice to restore health and balance to the human energy system, and so beneficial to every human, regardless of religious preference, spiritual pursuits, or scientific degrees of study. This is because it is of benefit to humans as a species, and so transcends culture, race, gender or any other way that humans choose to differentiate themselves from one another.

While this pure, energy vibration is a natural addition to the field of Energy Medicine, it does not mean that all Reiki professionals are Energy Medicine practitioners, or need to be. Reiki can, and does, stand-alone quite well.

THE APERTURE OF ENERGY

Understanding how energy works can help one achieve goals shared by many spiritual aspirants. This includes going beyond the constructs that limit us to living within created realities, to understand the whole of experience and what is possible as a human.

As everything is energy, it is the natural starting point for understanding the greater world we are a part of, what makes up the totality of a human being, and what defines experience. The answers to these questions, however interesting, lie beyond the scope of this book. However, they are mentioned here to convey that by understanding the simple truth that everything is energy, including you, and that you co-exist with other subtle and gross energies in a shared environment, you are constantly affecting one another, and the whole. When this is accepted and understood, experience can be viewed through an impersonal aperture. This new vantage point frees us up and encourages us to place importance upon the experience of life itself and on the quality of experience we allow in our lives, instead of the mundane aspects we imagine are important and use to define us.

This constitutes an enormous shift, where you can start to care for and nurture the experience of life you are partaking in, instead of defending the details of a life lived thus far. When this occurs, you will naturally seek out ways to create greater ease in your life by extending your understanding of the self-care that is required to live a freer, happier life.

To do this well, means starting our journey by accepting that there is more to us than what is met by our eyes. The discussion that follows includes topics on subtle, human anatomy that is commonly spoken and written about in a spiritual context. This limits the accessibility of information to only a small number of people desiring a spiritual experience. Even then, the information provided to this smaller, albeit attentive, audience, offers little to no explanation on how the human energy system works. So by stepping back, and discussing the subtle anatomy in terms of Energy Medicine, with a focus on Reiki, the information becomes immediately accessible and usable to a greater audience; which when used and practiced, can provide a deepening of understanding of how our parts come together and work as a whole. The reason this is important, and why I have spent the time and effort unpuzzling the puzzle and bringing this lost information back to a larger audience, is because in the effort to protect it or to control it, humans lost their understanding of Reiki, and so were robbed of their choice to use it.

The Human Bodies

The human form is made up of many parts that are commonly referred to as "bodies". Different traditions call these bodies by different names. Although there is some differentiation among these bodies, they, with the exception of one, work together and are inter-related. Generally speaking, these bodies are physical, auric, mental, psychic and astral. Some traditions and schools may offer an expanded or more descriptive list, or call some by different names. However, if we leave things to generalities and within the scope of Reiki, this explanation is complete and sufficient without taking us too far into tangents.

Reiki works directly on two of these bodies, the physical and auric. Reiki does this by restoring balance and making mild repairs where needed, which is effectively bringing together what has come apart through the daily wear and tear of living life. While Reiki works directly on two of the five bodies listed, it affects and influences the other bodies. Its influence, however, is limited, in that the Reiki vibration does not have the specialized nature required to bring change to ailments, illnesses or imbalances that have originated in those other bodies. This is an important distinction that lends insights and provides a framework for understanding the benefits and limitations of Reiki[5].

THE AURIC BODY

All living things have an energy system that includes an aura and chakra system. For the purposes of the study of Reiki, this discussion is limited to the human aura, and solely within the scope of Reiki.

The aura is the energy field that surrounds and protects the human body. The aura protects the subtle anatomy of the human body much like the skin protects the gross anatomy of the skeletal structure and internal organs of the body. The skin is a biologically gross form of protection for the human body, and the aura is an energetically subtle form of protection.

The chakra system is a series of energy vortexes that help to regulate the energy system of a human being and is part of the subtle anatomy that is the aura. There are many chakra points throughout the human body. However, in this discussion, we will focus on the seven major chakra areas that are shown to exist throughout the center of the human body.

As a Reiki student, the positions you learn to apply Reiki to correspond to these major chakra points. These major chakras points, and the minor ones found throughout the feet, are used as the primary distribution system by which Reiki is delivered to the whole of the human body.

Of special note, Reiki alone cannot repair damage done or distortions made to the chakras. The reason for this is that

---

[5] The next chapter goes into great detail in its discussion of the benefits and limitations of Reiki.

these types of injuries or imbalances are not caused through daily wear and tear, and are generally caused by some form of trauma. As such, other, subtler, healing vibrations within the Energy Medicine toolbox, can be used to remedy, repair and restore balance, and are often used along side of Reiki.

HOW THE REIKI VIBRATION DIFFERS FROM OTHERS

There are many natural, healing energy vibrations used in the field of Energy Medicine and by Natural Healers throughout the world. Different vibrations effect different bodies to provide remedy to ailments, imbalances, illness and injury. While knowledge of how to use these vibrations effectively requires study and knowledge of subjects highlighted at the start of the chapter, Reiki can be used immediately, as part of a daily self-care practice, after an attunement is completed.

There are many ways that Reiki differs from the host of natural, healing energies used in the world today. Our discussion will focus on three that truly distinguish Reiki from the others.

Firstly, in the world of natural healing, Reiki is considered a closed system because its purity cannot be manipulated by outside interference. This means that the mental or emotional state of the Reiki Practitioner, either of higher, purer quality or lower, poorer quality, does not affect the Reiki vibration. Some natural, healing vibrations, in order to work effectively, require a meditative state or another form of manipulation to work. This means the effectiveness of the vibration will depend greatly on the skill of the healer, the depth of training received, and the personal control and level of indifference obtained to heal. The use of these vibrations then, would fall into the category of advanced care, not self-care. Because Reiki does not require a meditative state, incantation spoken, or anything other than a cupped Reiki hand to work, Reiki is safe to use at home with family and friends.

This gently helps us transition into the second point that makes Reiki different, which is its accessibility. Reiki is immediately accessible and among the most widely known and taught of all healing vibrations. To receive information, and the ability to become a channel of Reiki, requires no pre-requisite knowledge of energy or human anatomy, and is easily taught and delivered through the attunement process, which is a ritual and short in duration. This differentiates Reiki from other healing vibrations that require years of tutelage and practice to become proficient.

The problem this creates, however, is misunderstanding about the vibration, and what is possible through its use and practice. In the absence of this understanding, Reiki can be, and often is, incorrectly described and used, which results in its benefits being overpromised and therefore found to under-deliver. When this happens the value and effectiveness of Reiki becomes questioned as it is expected to bring about a result that it was not designed to deliver. The example that follows helps to illustrate this point.

If you are using a hammer to try to loosen and remove a nut from a bolt, and have been taught to believe that a hammer is the correct tool to use to loosen and remove a nut from a bolt, you may very quickly become distrustful of hammers and disheartened by the level of difficulty and ineffectiveness of the hammer to perform the task at hand. Imagine again if this caused you to feel that hammers were useless and didn't do what they were promised to do. This is what has happened with many in regards to Reiki. It has either been subjugated as a meaningless therapy, or something that sort of works, but is not consistent. However, this could not be further from the truth because Reiki is incredibly consistent and powerful when used in the correct way, and for its correct purpose, just as a hammer is exceptional at placing a nail into the wall or removing a nail embedded into a piece of wood. In this capacity the hammer is effective and consistent.

The final point of differentiation is in regard to Reiki within an advanced-care practice. In most advanced-care practices, Reiki is used as one of many tools and it is shown much reverence. Many Energy Medicine Practitioners who are also Reiki Master Teachers, consider Reiki the simplest, purest, most solid, and robust healing system on the planet. This distinction is made because Reiki can be used alone or in conjunction with other healing vibrations without those other vibrations changing or altering the purity of Reiki, or Reiki altering them. In this capacity there is no equal. It is for this reason that Reiki is often used by Energy Medicine Practitioners together with other vibrations, because it provides a strong foundation for other subtler healing vibrations to work. To be clear, the use of Reiki is not required when using other healing vibrations or modalities. Using it or not is at the discretion of the Practitioner or Healer. However, in practice, using Reiki alongside other healing vibrations has been shown to consistently benefit and further support the client receiving healing.

OPEN TO SKEPTICISM

What makes the practice of Energy Medicine, like Reiki, open to skepticism is that much of what is used and understood is unseen and cannot be sufficiently measured by current research technology. Part of the progression in Modern Science today is in the development of instrumentation that can perceive and study subtler energies like the human aura, which science calls a biofield. These new technologies are beginning to change the way science looks at the whole of a human being, and is helping to bring this awareness to a wider audience.

However, even with greater awareness, there is still no way to prove to yourself or to another, what illness, injury or ailment you saved yourself from having to experience through a consistent practice of Reiki. This is equally true for brushing your teeth. While research and modern technology have proven that brushing your teeth on a consistent and regular basis is essential for good oral health, there is no way to prove, with complete certainty, what regular dental self-care saved you from experiencing or not. In fact, even with the best practice of personal dental hygiene, you may still require a root canal or have your wisdom teeth removed. Does that mean you failed, or that your dental care was incomplete? No. What it suggests instead is that occasionally more is required than tooth brushing alone to keep the mouth, jaw and gums in optimal health.

This back door that leads to the land of skepticism, cannot be destroyed and so is best avoided. The reason it cannot be destroyed is because it is a part of a mental process that also serves a valuable purpose; our natural desire to question things. However, it is best avoided because skepticism itself infers the existence of assumptions that pre-empt, or get in the way, by influencing experience before experience has taken place. It infers the person has "made-up his or her mind" about something and so it must be "proved" or "disproved" before the thing has been experienced. When this happens, the starting point of the individual is that experience is perceived in only one of the bodies, the mental body, and is so limited. What this means is a skeptical mind or point of view is a limited one that interferes with our ability to fully experience and know something. It is only by remaining open and allowing experience to be perceived through the whole body and all its senses, that you can truly become informed. I will take this one step further to say a skeptical mind or point of view is a protective one, designed to control the limits of reality accepted. A naturally inquisitive mind is open to experience and accepts the level of reality its experience can attain.

It is with this reminder that I end the section. The mind is a wonderful and valued tool that interprets human experience. The civilized world has misused this tool over the course of our time on earth, giving it more and more to do. This was done because it gave civilized humans a sense of control over their lives. What was forgotten was that the mind mostly interprets. The mind does not hear sound, see color, feel rain as it falls and touches the skin, but it interprets the experience and so provides a way to understand and explain it. Reiki is a vibration and so the mind cannot feel it, your body can and does, your mind then interprets the feeling and provides you with language to describe it.

REIKI IN ENERGY MEDICINE PRACTICE

In the clinic I co-founded we often start clients on a series of regular Reiki sessions before using subtler energy vibrations. There are many reasons for this.

First, it is a natural starting point when you consider that the majority of the human population is not using Reiki regularly to strengthen and re-balance, so we are starting the healing process with a compromised energy system. In this way, it is used to stabilize the client to make our work together easier and more effective. This could be likened to the way a medical doctor might start with an IV drip to ensure proper and adequate hydration, or a dentist who may first need to brush or floss the patient's teeth before starting any advanced work.

Second, Reiki is the best vibration for helping someone to relax well and deeply. Relaxation is key to human health and recovery, because it initiates our natural and innate healing abilities. It is when we are truly relaxed that true healing can take place.

Third, we use Reiki consistently, and in conjunction with other vibrations as treatment progresses, because it provides a strong foundation for other vibrations to work when those vibrations are necessary to affect change.

Lastly, we found that incorporating Reiki as a first step, and then as a platform to do advanced healing treatments, offers a complete and steady pace from which to take the person from imbalance, illness, injury or disease, to health. A slower, steadier pace helps the mind accept the changes that have occurred to restore health and well-being. By doing this we acknowledge that it is challenge to the mind, and to the sensibility of modern-day humans to accept immediate change, especially when recovering from a significant problem. While most people can accept that this is true of most, few will accept that this is also true of them. But as any Reiki Professional and Energy Medicine Practitioner will likely tell you, it is as important to get the mind to accept the restoration of health, as it is to restore it.

FOUR

THE BENEFITS &
LIMITATIONS OF REIKI

This discussion is among the most important in the study of Reiki today. It is where the most information is lacking, and where there is information, it is often incomplete or confusing. The reason for this is easier to see when you consider that contradictions are ever-present when you approach the study of Reiki in a linear manner.

As stated in an earlier chapter, many well-meaning people unknowingly make the mistake of overpromising, and under delivering on Reiki to themselves, and to others. The result of which leaves Reiki underappreciated for what it does do, and credited for things it doesn't do. This is not a fault of the Reiki vibration; rather, it is the result of people trying to understand it and create value for it as a practice to others.

There are many reasons for misunderstanding, most however, stem from the fact that Reiki is both effective at what it does do, while also offering benefits and support in areas where it does not offer direct remedy. In this way, the benefits of using Reiki are like waves, rippling out and improving processes in areas it does not directly influence or affect change in. While on the one hand this can be viewed as a wonderful benefit, it also helps to explain one of its perceived limitations.

One example of this is Reiki being confused as a meditative practice, which it is not. However, it does relax the body, and that aids and deepens meditation. While a deeper meditative practice may be desired by some, and so regarded as a benefit, if it is credited for and promoted as a meditative practice, it may cause others to dismiss Reiki, especially if they are not interested, or place value, on a meditative practice. This is just one of the reasons why it is important to offer as much clarity on what Reiki does, what it does not do, and to provide as much detail as possible about its benefits and its limitations.

The ultimate goal of course, is to reverse the trend of people who have received Reiki attunements that never, or rarely use Reiki, and to open the practice up to all people, as a practice every human can benefit from. To begin to do this successfully, we must stop selling Reiki as a cure all, or say it does things it does not do. To avoid this, gain a greater understanding of the vibration itself, and to, in a sense, re-introduce Reiki, let's get into the details.

GENERALLY SPEAKING

Generalities are brilliant when trying to explain things from a macro (general) point of view. However, it should always be noted that generalities often change when you start to apply them in a micro (specific) context. In an effort to provide the best foundation of information on Reiki, I will speak in generalities. In doing so, you will then have a solid framework that you can then start to apply specifics to.

Reiki works on the physical and auric bodies to repair and restore balance where imbalances have been created by the wear and tear of living in natural, and increasingly unnatural, environments. Natural environments consist of untouched land and open spaces that flow within the natural rhythms of planetary relationships. Unnatural environments include human-made landscapes, structures, urban/suburban areas, and interpersonal human relationships that place societal norms of acceptable behavior and influence over the natural rhythms of the human experience.

Humans are affected each day by these unseen forces, and as they are unseen, we generally end up attributing the affect they have on our lives to the interactions we have with the people, situations and circumstances of our lives. I will speak more about the mental process humans' use for understanding health and interpreting life events in greater detail later in this chapter. In the meantime, I will simply point out that because our mind has limited information and understanding, it is inaccurate and incomplete in its assessment and conclusions, more than it is correct.

To illustrate, imagine for a moment if all scientific information regarding how our planet and its weather patterns are influenced by its relationship to the sun and moon were lost, or worse, not accepted. Still, as a species, we would work tirelessly to understand the weather and to find ways to protect and prepare ourselves for its changes. And we would succeed in coming up with answers and processes for accommodating our daily lives, whatever the weather would bring. But, we would not have the best and most complete information, because things we don't know or don't accept would not be part of our consideration set, so we are left doing the best with the information we have, or are willing to accept. This practice leaves us vulnerable to unknowns, which is always the case, except many unknowns, certainly the ones discussed in this chapter, are known and can be now included in your understanding of general health and well-being. That, generally speaking, is the wonder and success of Reiki.

When I am seeing a client in my practice, more often than not, I will explain that while we may start with Reiki, Reiki alone will be insufficient to correct their problem. Going back to dental comparisons, Reiki can be, and should be, thought of more like an essential daily self-care practice, in the same way tooth brushing is. Through its regular and consistent use you can readily expect to save time, money, and drastically minimize the potential for pain and illness in the mouth that can, if left untreated, cause problems known and unknown within the body. With that said, if you are going to the dentist for anything more than a regular check-up, advanced tools and techniques are likely required to provide remedy to your immediate problem. Your dentist however, will still encourage tooth brushing on a regular basis and will likely do so by providing you with the parting gift of a new toothbrush, if not a tube of their favorite most trusted brand of toothpaste.

In the same way, if you are coming to see a Reiki and/or Energy Medicine Professional for an acute or chronic problem,

Reiki is likely not the best or appropriate medicine to correct the nature of that problem. In fact, a good general rule to follow is if you have received a diagnosis for an aliment, illness, condition or injury, Reiki alone is not going to bring about change. It may help to provide you with temporary relief from symptoms and boost your natural healing abilities, but it will not help you correct or change the diagnosis. Any promises that it will are empty promises that will ultimately end in failure. Reiki is not a vibration designed and created for this purpose. There are others that do that. Reiki does what I have started and will continue to state throughout the book, and it really is that straightforward and simple. But to advance and to help integrate that understanding let's review and go deeper.

Human are made up of a combination of subtle and gross energies. Most illnesses, diseases and imbalances begin in the subtler energy bodies before increasing to a point where they embed themselves in our gross anatomy. That all sounds a bit extreme and in some cases can be, but there are more examples of smaller more inconvenient illnesses or ailments than there are extreme ones. The key to correcting them is to catch them early before an imbalance can embed itself and create illness. While Reiki does this very well on imbalances in the physical and auric bodies, Reiki does not work on ailments, illness and/or imbalances that have originated in the mental, psychic or astral bodies. It will also not cure illness already embedded within the body, and it will not be able restore balance to areas within the body where mental or emotional blocks are causing disease. These ailments require other healings energies administered by a well trained, and an extraordinarily well balanced, Energy Medicine professional or Healer. In all these cases however, continued and consistent use of Reiki will make everything easier and will help keep the person affected more comfortable.

Reiki has no contraindications known, or experienced in any recorded case found. It is not known to ever cause discomfort, regardless of the number of symptoms experienced. It works with medications of all cultural practices, with all religions and spiritual faiths, and with all natural, energy vibrations. This is because Reiki is as natural and necessary to the human energy system as water is to the human body.

Home Remedy & Self-Care

As children we are taught through a series of life events how to care for our bodies and for our general well-being. Of course the quality of that teaching varies and is largely dependent upon the quality of teachers we had, their personal commitment to self-care, and then later how that shaped our own personal commitment. Even among the best levels of self-care taught, still most are not aware or taught how to take care of the human energy field. That changes with Reiki.

The Reiki vibration is to the human energy system, what brushing and flossing is to your mouth: a means to provide good health, preventative in nature, and leaves a sense of general well-being to the whole. It is effective in this way because it helps to make necessary repairs to the body and auric field, as both are affected by the influences and imbalances within a given environment. This is done through a knitting together of what may have been torn ever slightly apart through the daily wear and tear of life. I like to think of it like cleaning and mending a shirt that has come through a busy bustling city, which as a result of its day becomes full of debris, and in most cases may have a tear or stain on its sleeve.

While some people live in tranquil settings, most live in busy, bustling areas; what is key is not to be misled by appearances. What is of greater importance to understand is the speed at which you move through the world. For even a seemingly tranquil sub-urban area can be wrought with energetic imbalances when you consider the impact and affect our daily interactions have on our general well-being. So then, depending on the relationships you have with the people in your life, any external setting, tranquil or not, can feel at times like a war zone.

If you have ever felt that coming out of the DMV (Driver and Motor Vehicle Department) was like being put through a sieve, or notice that you often feel drained after grocery shopping, or many times feel that you can't get out of your Mother's or friend's house fast enough, it is because on some level, perhaps even on many levels, you are aware that the energy of these places, people and the daily activities you are engaged in are affecting the general, health, balance and ease of your human being.

For most, these experiences will result in the person feeling they need to get home, secure in the knowledge that home is a place of respite and where one can relax. This however, is not all that is needed to mend and rebalance from the day. If it were, people would not feel the need to use alcohol, television, prescription drugs, food or even sex to help them relax. In fact, while each of these things may help a human achieve a momentary level of relaxation, they all come with the cost of other side effects, which in and of themselves create imbalance within the human bodies.

Relaxation then, is the foundation on which your self-care regime is built, and without a good and strong foundation, any and all self-care treatments will be limited in its ability to provide ease, improve health and restore balance. Its value cannot be underemphasized, as it is a necessary part, and a precursor to, your body's natural healing process. It is for this reason that most discussions on Reiki start by describing it as a means to provide natural and deep relaxation. Once it is understood that the body's ability to relax on demand, and the quality of relaxation that can be achieved on demand, directly influences the body's ability to heal well and efficiently, the need for better information regarding how this can be achieved becomes of greater importance. When this previously unknown information becomes known and understood, the desire to provide deeper and more sustainable levels of self-care becomes naturally sought after.

Reiki is among the most effective and efficient vibrations to bring about natural relaxation. This is because although it works predominately on only two bodies, it works in harmony with all the bodies that make up the human body, so there is no conflict between them. This is a key point to highlight, for this is not true of most modalities used to established relaxation. Non-Reiki modalities usually work on one of the bodies, but at the expense or against one of the others. The result then is experienced as a modest sense of relaxation achieved while the method is being used, but once the method is stopped, the sense of relaxation begins to fade.

Reiki is different and its effects are cumulative. Examples that highlight these cumulative effects include, our emotional state and reactions to things becomes more balanced, our ease in getting to sleep is better and our quality of sleep is improved. Best of all, our ability to relax on demand is restored. When this happens our body returns to the natural ebb and flow of action and relaxation.

From relaxation to general health, Reiki can provide immediate remedy to common bumps and bruising as well as general aches and pains. Reiki can help people recover with greater speed and efficiency from surgery, illness and injury. I offer a very general list here because while there are many things Reiki will do well for every person that uses it, each person has a complexity of thoughts, emotions, and karmas that shape, and are shaped, by the life experiences and choices made. All of which affect our health, ease of being, state of mind, and overall balance.

While the overall benefits received by Reiki are the same for every human, the remedies it provides will always be limited to the scope of its use. Effectively this means that while every person will receive the same benefits using Reiki, Reiki will not always bring about remedy desired even when two seemingly similar people are experiencing similar symptoms.

The appearance of similar symptoms, even when presented in what appears to be similar individuals can be deceiving. This is because causes creating symptoms, that at first view appear to be the same, can in fact be different. Reiki will bring about remedy when the cause of the problem is in one of the bodies Reiki works on directly and will not provide remedy if the cause is outside of those bodies and so outside of its sphere of influence. While I realize that on the surface this may be confusing, at a deeper level its not. I will give an example to help illustrate.

Two women suffer from the pain and discomfort that can accompany the monthly menstrual cycle. Woman A uses Reiki each month because it is brilliant in taking care of her menstrual cramps, while Woman B finds no relief from her menstrual cramps when using Reiki. The reason for this is that the imbalance effecting Women A is in one of the bodies that Reiki provides remedy to, while the imbalance affecting Woman B is not. In this way Reiki can be a brilliant tool for both women. For even though Reiki has brought about change in Woman A and not Woman B, Woman B is now sure that the cause of her discomfort is in another area, which can help her find the healing and remedy she needs to effect the change she desires. Furthermore, while Reiki did not provide direct remedy to Woman B, Reiki still helped her relax and helped to energize her in other areas, which may make the pain easier to bear while she seeks out another remedy. In both cases, it is clear that Reiki works, but that its work is limited to the scope of influence it has on the bodies that make up the human body.

The following illustrates a modern Western medical treatment to further our understanding of how Reiki can treat similar symptoms but achieve different results depending on cause or origination of ailment. Regardless of how you feel about antibiotics, they are effective in killing bacteria that affect human health. However, antibiotics are only successful in treating ailments created through a bacterial infection and will not work on viral infections. In this way, if two people report symptoms from an upper respiratory infection, one caused by a bacterial infection and the other caused by a viral infection, the antibiotics will only work to provide relief to one and not the other. However, Reiki, unlike antibiotics, has no negative side effects and while it may not bring remedy to ailments outside of its scope, it will still provide relaxation, and in that way supports what will provide a more permanent remedy.

So, if through its use you find that Reiki is not alleviating a symptom, it is not because Reiki does not work. It is because the cause of that symptom resides in one of the other bodies that Reiki does not directly work on. When this occurs, a good general rule to follow is that your need for balance and healing exceeds that achieved through self-care practices. In these instances, seek treatment and remedy from other sources, for doing so when needed is also a measure of self-care. In fact, seeking healing or advanced care outside of your self-care practice will be necessary on occasion, and is something to be expected either as a source of remedy from ailments or injury, as a means to provide greater clarity and balance, or in the way of a check-up to be sure small things are not being missed.

So expect to need advanced care, but don't allow the advanced care you seek to take the place of, or to interrupt, your self-care practice, because they are two different things. Remember that in the same way seeing a Dentist does not relieve you of the daily responsibility of brushing and flossing, seeking advanced care for ailments, injuries and illness does not take the place of your daily need and practice of Reiki. Additionally, as you would never expect a Dentist to ask you to stop brushing or flossing your teeth while you are under their care, a healer of any kind should never ask you to stop using Reiki while you are under his or hers. If they do, I would ask them if they know Reiki and if they don't, I would take the time to show it to them and to explain how and why you use it. If after your explanation and demonstration they continue to ask you to stop, I would encourage you ask them why, and consider getting a second opinion. This is because Reiki is as pure, natural, and as vital to the human energy system as water is to the human body, and like water, has no known contraindications.

IN PROFESSIONAL PRACTICE

As a Reiki professional, I view my role as one that provides my clients with Reiki, information, and a forum to discuss the level of self-care they give to themselves. This discussion starts by reviewing the grosser aspects of self-care and then moves to the subtler. An example of a gross aspect of self-care would include the amount of water a person drinks a day, where the subtler aspects would include how kind they are to themselves in any given situation, and whether or not they place the needs of the other people in their lives above their own. All levels of discussion are at the complete discretion of the clients.

As most people without a regular Reiki practice are unknowingly riddled with imbalances, the effects of the initial treatments are felt fairly immediately. I am clear to explain that Reiki is used as a means to help clients recover from illness or injury because it naturally boosts their body's natural healing abilities. I further make the distinction that while self-care Reiki can do this, the benefit of seeing a Reiki professional is in his or her advanced knowledge of the vibration and the clarity their impartiality provides. It is the clarity found through impartiality that is of remarkable mention, particularly if someone is healing from a significant illness, injury or ailment. For in those cases, it is difficult not to worry, or to have the mind create scenarios and explanations that can, and often do, slow down the body's natural course of recovery.

In many scenarios, but not all, we find that we will come to a limit and have done as much as we can at the moment with Reiki. It is at this point then that the use of other healing vibrations can be used to help the process along, where and if we have hit a plateau. It is important here to note that often the plateau was reached and then identified through the successful use of Reiki, which took us to the point of revealing that something more was required. In practice, I continue to use Reiki as a foundation and alongside other healing vibrations.

Following nearly all types of sessions, Reiki or otherwise, I often ask clients if they have received a Reiki attunement. If they have, I will ask them to demonstrate how they give themselves Reiki before leaving the session. I do this to check hand position and to support them in their daily practice, as people over time can get naturally lazy and their cupped Reiki hand position can start to fall flat. I encourage each person to continue their self-care practice and ask them if, or where, they feel they are failing short by forgetting to use Reiki. I use this as an opportunity to explore why, instill more information, and to help answer questions or provide insight into what may be holding them back.

What I make clear to students and clients is that the advanced care you receive from a Reiki professional should prove to boost your self-care practice. Reiki students of all levels, including that of Reiki Master Teacher, can benefit greatly from periodically receiving sessions from another Reiki professional. Equally, Reiki professionals should never feel threatened and as a result fail by missing the opportunity to encourage the self-care practice of their clients and students; for both boost and support the other, and without each, progression of the practice and its place in human health becomes diminished.

How the Mind Affects Healing

As it stands, it is part of the mind's job to provide us with explanations and a dialogue to share our experiences. The mind's ability to do this part of its job is limited by what it knows and accepts as reality. It is then within the bounds of a self-contained consideration set that the mind explains and defines experience, pain, illness, behavior, and anything else that is required. These explanations are subjective and filter through the collection of experiences that make up and are aligned with a world-view deemed acceptable by society first, and then by our personality.

In terms of our health and well-being, the explanations offered to our conscious mind are incorrect and incomplete if they are absent of an acceptance and understanding that the human body and its experience is influenced on a daily basis by many unseen energies. In the absence of this acceptance, internal prejudices prevail and cloud our judgment, and it is in this cloud, that we get lost. For the prevailing wisdom is that the mind is too big to be understood, which is not the case. Its complexity is self-induced and we have built upon it consistently as long as we as a species have existed on the planet. This complexity, or turning in on itself, is a result of us asking more and more from it as a way to control and create realities we can live with. While the next section steps quietly outside of our Reiki discussion to provide insights into how and why this happened, it is done in the hope of helping you understand how the mind affects everything human, and that includes our use of Reiki.

The Mind on its Own

As discussed in an earlier chapter, there are many bodies that make up the human body. These bodies, identified earlier as physical, auric, mental astral, and psychic, were all originally created to work together and affect one another in most, if not all, aspects of human existence.

Over time and in many ways, humans have corrupted the planet's natural environment. These produced countless changes in the way humans live, which then influenced and affected human experience by creating more and different levels of imbalance. These imbalances then grew and ultimately caused the separation of the mental body from the others. This separation was the result of us consistently using the mind in a way it was not designed or intended to be used. The problem with us doing this is that we didn't accept or understand the cost of it then, and we still don't now, because we continue to do this.

A balanced mind is one that accepts experience and archives it in memory, organizes it as learning, categorizes and prioritizes it based on tasks required for well-being (such as self-care), sorts it by importance in terms of our biological and social welfare and provides language to it, so that it can be shared. As a part of our evolution as a species, we unbalanced the mind when we began using it to help us cope by interpreting reality and justifying actions taken within this new world we were creating and forging life in. We then found that the interpretation of reality wasn't enough. In fear and a growing need to feel in control, we asked it to do more by creating false or imagined realities that were easier to accept, and would provide a mental state we call peace of mind. This desire and need for a false sense of security, or a point of view that chooses to see the world as it "should be" instead of how it is, required us as a species to disconnect our mind from the other bodies, and so became the dominating force defining perception. The reason disconnection is essential to living in this way and was inevitable, is because the human form is biologically bound to respond to reality or, the world as it is. To experience the "should be" version, the mind must dominate the whole of experience and in so doing bypass the natural ebb and flow of our being, which is experiencing through the body by feeling ourselves individually and as part of a shared environment.

The undue and constant stress of using the mind to create multiple, and simultaneously running realities, has forced us to make adjustments in the way humans learn and process information. When our mental body separated and became the dominant tool used, we limited learning to a mental function. While the mind can define, organize, anticipate, judge, catalog, describe, sort, argue, and do other truly useful things that help us, the mind is unable to experience, so depending on the mind alone leaves us stilted in our ability to truly learn. To truly know and learn any thing, the learning of facts must be accompanied by experience and incorporated into the whole. The mind alone cannot do this, and we have forgotten how tactile learning has made it possible for us to do many of the things we do each day, like drive a car, or play an instrument, or understand how to use a computer.

Mastery of any subject is accompanied by an expansive perspective and vision that sees how the parts make up the whole, and how the whole influence the parts. But learning through the mind alone limits our focus by defining things in starts and stops; such as, here is where this starts, and there is where that stops. The bodies that make up the human form and the systems within it do not work this way. The remaining bodies work together, constantly flowing within and influencing one another. So, to understand the human body and the many ways with which to provide healing to it, it may be helpful to think of water.

No description of water, technical, lyrical or otherwise, can take the place of your experience of it; the feeling of being submersed in it, of having it flow through your fingers, of taking it in to quench a thirst. Water is to be experienced, if it is to be known. As a species, we are at its mercy. Despite our attempts to control it, route it, and measure it, we are still in a constant state of submission to its greater whims. Too much water and we drown, not enough and we die. Our bodies and our lives are always in search of balance when it comes to water, and despite the amount of data and information we think we know about it, it remains, like us, a mystery.

Arguably, the most notable change and affect of the mind's dominance, is that it has resulted in humans feeling less, projecting more, and losing the ability to know the difference between them or when this is happening.

What I describe here is the difference between a person *feeling* happy and a person projecting happiness. Feeling happy is a bodily sensation and as it is experienced, it is undeniable. Projecting happiness is when a person receives information that society has taught them they should be happy about, and so they project happiness by engaging in behaviors that are consistent with what society has taught them mirror happiness. In the West it is more often the case than not, that the description of how a person feels differs from how the person actually feels. This happens when a person is living in his or her head, so to speak, and is disconnected from their emotions and feelings. This is a learned behavior that is taught to children and reinforced by society throughout adult life.

The key, to restoring balance and improving overall health, is in knowing how you feel. To be as clear as possible, this means feeling through the body, not interpreting, assessing, projecting or describing feeling, which has become the accepted norm in civilized societies. Acute symptoms such as pain will bypass created realities and mental projections, but chronic pain, unless severe, may not. Additionally, smaller symptoms can be easily missed as you reassure yourself that everything is all right and that you are tired or run-down because you worked all day. This is not to say that working all day will not make you tired or run-down, but unless you are aware how you feel, which is different then how you think you feel, your exhaustion could be a symptom or caused by an imbalance that can be remedied by Reiki or by another advanced-care treatment.

By understanding the greater scope of what we as humans are exposed to and influenced by, we give the mind more information to consider as we task it with providing answers. The mind loves this and it's a natural part of its job. So stop asking the mind to experience, which is something it cannot do, and start experiencing the greater world around you and your place in it. You can start the process by engaging the five major senses. This is very different than allowing them to run on automatic pilot. When they are engaged, you will likely be surprised by the amount of information they provide. Then ask your mind to list them, catalog them, and construct questions about them. These are just some of the tasks the mind does well and is part of what it was naturally created to do.

It is helpful to remember that you cannot live without the mind and that the mind is a precious part of the human form. The fault then, is not with the mind, but how we misuse it. With this information, change is possible and while Reiki does not work directly on the mental body, the use of Reiki can help you re-establish your connection to feeling the body, re-engage the senses and explore the benefits inherent in tactile learning.

Using Reiki is a good first step. It is tactile. It requires a specific hand position and its experience is felt, it cannot be projected. Receiving it will provide ease and a general sense of relaxation and calm. This is a bodily feeling, which is to say; it is a feeling that is felt through the body, not the mind.

FIVE

EMBARKING ON REIKI

Out of reverence for the oral tradition and the relationship between student and Master Teacher, I will not detail "how to" administer Reiki on yourself or others. Most books do this by including dozens of photographs of Reiki hands being laid upon various parts of the human body. The learning and practice of placing Reiki hands on yourself or someone else for the first time is special. It is you becoming part of an ancient initiation process that is only to be experienced through the instruction and aid of a carefully chosen Reiki Master Teacher. This ancient initiation process is called a Reiki attunement. Your Reiki Master Teacher who will perform the attunement will also instruct and guide you on how to use Reiki on yourself and others. It is then through practice that they may provide correction and additional as needed instruction, while you, the student, begins to feel for yourself Reiki flowing through your hands into your body or the body of another. To be clear, receiving the attunement ritual should be the beginning of your relationship with a Reiki Master Teacher, not the end.

For these reasons, over-the-internet or over-the-phone Reiki attunements, at any level, should be avoided. This is true no matter the qualifications being claimed by the Reiki Master Teacher offering the service. The reason for this is that a Reiki attunement will forever change and affect the energy and chakra system of your body. It would be wise then to give the same quality of careful consideration you give to your Reiki attunement that you would in deciding which doctor you would use to perform a minor surgical or dental procedure.

A Reiki attunement is safe, just as many small surgical procedures are safe when you work with someone who is uniquely qualified, and that you trust to do the best job possible. Ultimately, it is you that will live with the affects of your attunement, and so the responsibility is yours to find someone worthy of your confidence and trust in performing your Reiki attunement.

Finding a Reiki Master Teacher

It is recommended to start the process with an excitement about receiving a Reiki attunement and all it has to offer. If you do, you will do what comes naturally to you when looking for a good dentist or family doctor, which is to talk with the people you believe make good responsible choices about their self-care and seek guidance. Avoid making a choice merely on the words found in an advertisement. Advertisements should be like road signs. They should help point you in a direction where you can gather more information. Promises of quick attunements, or that multiple attunements can be done at one time or over the course of a weekend, should be avoided.

Most anyone can be attuned to Reiki Level I, and for the most part, Reiki Level I is all a person needs to provide them and their family with the level of self-care Reiki provides and the body requires. To go beyond Reiki Level I is something that is best done after the student has lived with and used Reiki for a considerable amount of time. I would consider that to be about a six-month period of consistent regular use.

GIVING TIME BETWEEN ATTUNEMENTS

Receiving a Reiki Level I attunement is like being given a new muscle. Using Reiki is using that muscle. Your new muscle, like all muscles, must be used consistently and as part of a regular practice for the muscle to build and grow. As the muscle builds, so will your energetic strength and your innate knowledge of Reiki. Additionally, the more you use your Reiki muscle, the more you will know for yourself if you wish to go further in your understanding of the practice to want to become a professional Reiki healer, or teach Reiki to others.

To be clear, a Reiki Level I attunement is all that is needed to provide self-care and general care to others. In the West, we imagine more is better and place importance on titles as a way to communicate proficiency, and worse still, mastery, of a subject. Mastery, however is not found in a title, it is acquired in practice and much of it. Rushing the process from student to Master comes at a cost. Receiving multiple attunements in short order over the Internet or over the course of a weekend workshop will provide you with tons of information, but it will leave you with very little knowledge or understanding of Reiki.

For most, this kind of pursuit results in the person rarely using what they learned, so the information is easily forgotten and becomes nothing more than a memory of something done at a weekend event some time ago. For what cannot be taught, provided or instilled through an Internet course or weekend workshop of artificially expedited advanced attunements, is reverence. Real and unbending reverence, like knowledge, requires practice and direct personal experience.

While multiple attunements may successfully embed Reiki Master symbols, and through it information into your energy body, it will not make you a knowledgeable Reiki Master teacher. That takes time and practice. In the same way, if a Martial Arts Master decided he or she could give the information and standing of Black Belt to a student over the course of a weekend, it would in no way give the student the ability, bodily knowledge and coordination to embody the information and be a practicing Black Belt. The same is true in the progression and practice of Reiki.

I have seen Reiki Level I students dedicated and pure in the practice mistaken for Reiki Masters by Reiki Master Teachers. This is because the knowledge of Reiki the Reiki Level I person embodied through their regular and consistent practice. I have been one of those students who, at Reiki Level II, was approached by a Master and asked for training. I offer these experiences to emphasize that this is not something that can or should be rushed.

A master of anything is not merely a title that can be given. It is a practice and a dedication to a practice that takes time, commitment and then more practice. Promises that indicate otherwise are empty promises to short cuts that bypass opportunity. For Reiki is no different than the martial arts, or music, or literature, or any other course of study that produces a Master. Masters on those subjects are made over time through consistent practice and cannot be rushed over the course of a weekend.

So if your aim is to go beyond learning the self-care of Reiki and into professional practice, or become a teacher of Reiki and an initiator into its tradition, consider an alternate path to receiving higher-level Reiki attunements once you have received your Reiki Level I. To do this well, find a Reiki Master Teacher you trust and feel confident has the energy and Reiki understanding necessary to give you a complete and well-executed attunement. Find a Reiki Master Teacher that you feel you can have a teacher/student relationship with over the long term, so that you may contact them and ask questions as the need arises and your practice progresses.

A Reiki Master Teacher committed to helping you attain a level of understanding that is embedded in the vibration itself and experienced through receiving and giving Reiki, will likely interview you to discuss the reasons you wish for a higher-level attunement. They will consider your commitment before offering you more information. The reason for this is found in the old proverb, 'you cannot pour water into a full cup'. And while the idea of more is better is deeply rooted into the culture of the Western educational system, Reiki knowledge cannot be fast-tracked, for if it is, it comes at the expense of understanding. In the world of Reiki, less is more.

Reiki Divided

Reiki has become a house divided within itself. Not entirely so, but on key points that have inadvertently led to misunderstandings in instruction and diluted the purity of its practice. This has left many people confused about what Reiki is and how to use it properly. Often these disagreements come down to perceived differences that have become established within the lineages. I use the word perceived because these are more preferences than differences, and are more imagined than real. They have, however, resulted in creating real differences in instruction that over the years downgraded Reiki and its place within self-care and advanced-care regimes.

As its oral tradition diminished, personal preferences of reigning Reiki Master Teachers surfaced, further diluting its ancient information. Some reasons for doing this were to legitimize Reiki and make it interesting within different cultural frameworks. While this explains what occurred and its result, it is only by returning to the purity and simplicity of the vibration that we can recapture what was lost. To do this well, judgment for its history, or for the choices of past leaders, is a waste of time.

Reiki is pure: people are not. Reiki Master Teachers are humans and so, imperfect and flawed. This is best not used as a form of judgment or division, but better understood as a means to bring things back together, which is something the pure vibration of Reiki does naturally.

The current division in Reiki can be found in three discussion points: Reiki hand position, derivations of practice taught, which I refer to as spin-offs, and whether a Reiki Master

Teacher teaches the value of, and requires, an adjustment period following an attunement, and for what length of time.

REIKI HANDS

Improper instruction and information regarding the effective Reiki hand position has found its way through every lineage and is now a subject of misunderstanding and division within the Reiki community.

To begin using Reiki, one must begin the initiation process of being attuned to the use of the vibration from a Reiki Master Teacher. This process prepares the energy system of a human to become a conduit of the vibration and to stream the vibration on demand. Once attuned, the student then needs to be instructed on how to "turn it on" to stream Reiki on demand. The cupped Reiki hand position is the "on" switch. When the person holds their hand in the Reiki cupped position, Reiki will naturally stream out of it. This is a distinction of note, because most students will wrongly assume that hand position is not important to the practice of Reiki or that is it less important than the attunement, but hand position is important because it is the "on" switch and your proficiency in using it properly will determine the flow of Reiki experienced.

A flat hand is what is often pictured in books and websites. A flat hand is not a conduit for Reiki to stream through. Reiki energy streams through a cupped hand. The best description I've heard to explain the cupped hand position comes from Tiffany Hunter, one of my Reiki Master Teachers. She says, "put your hand in a cupped position as if you were holding water and didn't want it to leak out." While I find this description initially produces an exaggeration of the cupped hand position, her logic for doing so is sound. For time and experience in working with hundreds of students has taught her that while a slight exaggeration of the cupped hand position may happen during instruction, in practice the hand will naturally become more relaxed and in so doing produces the optimal hand position for consistent and regular practice.

If an attuned individual is not using the proper hand position, they are not getting the proper flow of Reiki energy coming through. The good news is that if you are using an ineffective hand position, and so getting less from Reiki than you can be, all that can change in an instant. Simply change your hand position to the cupped Reiki position and feel the difference for yourself.

To know if you are using the correct hand position to yield the strongest Reiki or not, simply try it both ways; flat hand, and then cupped Reiki hand. If you don't feel the difference right away, don't worry, keep practicing and experimenting.

Also be aware that if you are accustomed to placing a flat hand on your chest and entering into a meditative state, then cupping your hand may feel awkward at first. If this occurs, it is because you're starting to change a habit. It does not mean you have to give up your flat hand meditation, it simply means that if you want to receive Reiki, you will also need to spend some time applying a cupped Reiki hand on or near your body.

I have worked with many students who have experimented by comparing the flattened hand position they were taught, with what is described here. In that time, I have never seen anyone claim that a flat palm produced more Reiki that the Reiki cupped hand position. In fact, every person I have seen try this for themselves has readjusted their practice to a cupped hand position and usually have done so with an exclamation like, "Wow!" This is because the cupped hand position will produce a strong Reiki vibration coming through and the other will not. This experimentation can be as fun as it is informative, and once you have received a Reiki attunement it is yours to enjoy.

REIKI SPIN-OFFS

There is one Reiki. Reiki is a vibration, and a simple practice was created to teach and to administer it. Adding symbols, levels of study, copyrights, or other healing techniques does not change, or alter the vibration of Reiki. This is the single greatest thing about Reiki. It is pure. Today there are many different type of healing systems that include the word Reiki in the name, that are not Reiki. In many cases these new healing systems were created by well meaning Reiki Master Teachers trying to make sense and progress the practice of Reiki by claiming unique or special knowledge of a new method that Reiki has evolved into. However, this has done more to set the understanding of the practice of Reiki back, than it has to progress it. It has done this by creating more confusion and spreading misinformation that promises levels of healing that Reiki was not created to achieve.

The creation of spin-offs of Reiki is a very human thing to do. As a species we are curious creatures that tend to complicate things we don't understand as a means to explain them. As mentioned earlier, judgment of such practices does nothing to help provide the clarity required to restore the understanding of the pure practice of Reiki. What will, however, is engaging the part of our nature that likes to take things apart to see how it works. For when it comes understanding Reiki, the natural place to start is by engaging the cupped Reiki hand, tuning in to how it feels, and how it is changing how you feel.

Avoid promises then, of supernatural experiences and light healing, if what you are looking for, is the healing qualities Reiki naturally provides. Supernatural concepts are easy to explain and sell, if you are willing, because they are mostly mental manipulations of experience designed to bring you into what is commonly referred to as an optimistic state of mind that temporarily alleviates crippling fears and daily worries. Some refer to this optimistic state of mind as the bliss state. While many seek this state and enjoy it for a time, it's temporary and so remains elusive because it is more of a mental manipulation than it is actual healing. What I describe here is the difference between actually *feeling* better, and the mental projection that mirrors what the mind perceives to be feeling better. The former is a bodily sense of ease that is accompanied by a greater overall sense and feeling of well-being, while the latter is not a feeling, but a state of mind.

It may be difficult to feel the difference between those two states at first, and to be successful in being able to consistently differentiate between the two; you have to really want to. If you do, then with practice you can become acutely aware between your mind feeling better and your body feeling better. Your mind can lie and make you believe you feel better at the expense of the body. The body cannot lie. When the body feels better, healing has taken place and health has improved.

ADJUSTMENT PERIOD TO FOLLOW

On the surface, the adjustment period following an attunement sounds like something that is separate from the attunement itself. On one hand it is, and on the other it isn't. The attunement itself is a ritual that is performed with you by a Reiki Master Teacher. The daily practice and restrictions of use that follow, as part of the requirements of the adjustment period, is where the student then supports their body into fully integrating the attunement received.

The adjustment period sets the foundation of the attunement, which makes the attunement as solid as possible. Not all Reiki lineages require or teach the value of an adjustment period following the attunement ritual. Of the ones that do, time period allotments will vary. For example, the lineage I am on requires and teaches the value of a 21-day adjustment period, while another Reiki Master Teacher I have worked with completed a 90-day adjustment period as part of his tutelage.

Without an adjustment period following the attunement, the attunement will still set, but will not be set on a solid foundation. While some may have no problems as a result of this, others may. Examples of problems may include feeling the flow of Reiki to be spotty and inconsistent, or the process of giving Reiki less than enjoyable. If this is the case, or if you have any problems following your Reiki attunement, talk with your Reiki Master Teacher right away and if you are still not satisfied, consider speaking to a Reiki Master Teacher on a lineage that requires an adjustment period. You have the right and the responsibility to ask as many questions as you need to regarding your attunement, its process and the lineage you are a part of or considering becoming a part of. Equally, if you are not satisfied with the answers you are getting, it is your right and responsibility to seek a second opinion. The current state of Reiki is that there is division in the ways it is taught, explained and performed. To know what is right and best for you, you will need to ask questions and to feel out what it right and best for you.

I can tell you I am deeply happy with, and have become enriched by, the adjustment period required and taught to me through the lineage I am a part of. I not only found it complete in accomplishing what it intended to, I feel it also gave me confidence in my practice. It did that by giving me the direct experience required to integrate the verbal instruction provided to me by my Reiki Master Teachers to turn it into knowledge. It also set the foundation for the personal commitment I would make, when I accepted and experienced first hand, that providing self-care to my energy is as important to my general health as the self-care I give to my physical body.

SIX

RECEIVING REIKI

In an earlier chapter it was explained that knowledge on any subject is achieved through the combination of two things: satisfying the mind's need for information and the body's need for direct experience. In this way, the first part of the book focuses on providing the former, while these remaining chapters focus on the latter.

It is here then, that our conversation shifts and expands from one of providing information on Reiki, to one that moves into the realm of experience. If you are attuned at any level, try reading this while also giving yourself Reiki and see if and how you experience Reiki, or the information provided, in a new or different way. This can and should be fun.

REIKI IS EVERYWHERE

The Reiki vibration is naturally plentiful on the planet and flows through every room and outdoor open space, like radio waves do. So then, if Reiki is plentiful on the planet and is here to help humans in the ways described above, then is everyone receiving Reiki with or without a Reiki attunement? The answer is yes, you are, and you have been since the moment you were born. It is the reason your body knows innately what to do with Reiki and how to use it. The problem is, that without being properly attuned you haven't been receiving enough of it and you haven't been able to use what you do receive efficiently.

The reason this is important is that there are countless energies on the planet that we come in contact with everyday. These energies have unseen but substantial effects on us. Within a natural environment, say a remote country setting or up on a mountain, the impact these energies have on us are less than in the unnatural environment of a city or a sub-urban area.

As populated areas grow in size and density, so too do the numbers of energies we come in contact with. These energies affect the human body. This is a growth trend that is not soon to change when as a species; we are easily seduced by the conveniences found in urban and sub-urban living. The result, however, is that these conveniences come at the expense of our bodies, which must contend with the impact and imbalances it creates within us. These imbalances, if not corrected, can build and progress from subtle imbalances in the human energy system into gross imbalances in the human form. Reiki is the naturally intended remedy to help the human energy system recover, repair, and rebalance from the effects environmental energies have on us.

Receiving a Reiki attunement changes that by supporting the body to use more of the natural Reiki vibration available on the planet. Receiving Reiki by self-administering it to yourself or by receiving it from another furthers the ability of the body to channel the vibration where it is needed most, and supports the body in using it efficiently and to your body's optimum.

MANY WAYS TO RECEIVE REIKI

With a Reiki attunement, Reiki can be self administered, given to you by a friend who is Reiki Level I attuned, or received as part of a formal Reiki Session by a Reiki professional. Receiving Reiki requires no ritual or regime. It can be as informal as you placing a cupped Reiki hand on your back while you stand in line at the grocery store to alleviate an aching back, placing your hands over your head for 10 minutes to relieve the temporary pain of a headache, or as formal as you taking the time to enjoy a full Reiki session given to yourself or received from a Reiki Practitioner.

Formal sessions given by a Reiki Level II, Master or Master Teacher are generally given in a serene setting. The person receiving the Reiki is usually either sitting comfortably or lying down. Both the person giving and the person receiving Reiki are fully clothed at all times and some relaxing music may be played. The Practitioner will then place their cupped Reiki hands directly on the physical body, or a few inches above, as they go through a series of set position points that start from the top of the head and proceed down to the feet.

Personally speaking, I usually work a few inches above the body, but whether you are working directly on the body or above it, if the person agrees to receive Reiki, they are receiving it in equal measure.

The Person Receiving Reiki is in Control

As part of the attunement process the person receiving the Reiki attunement is taught to provide Reiki through major points within the body. This includes the major chakra points, as well as minor ones located throughout the feet. While this is a brilliant practice and is thorough in nature, it does not replace your body's knowledge of itself and its awareness of where its needs are at all times.

What this means is that the body of the person receiving Reiki controls the flow and direction of Reiki as it enters into the body. If there is a pressing or immediate need, it will route the Reiki from where it is being received on the body to where the body needs it most. This is a bodily knowing, not a mental knowing. Your body knows best and you can trust it without hesitation.

Equally, the person receiving Reiki can decide if they will receive the Reiki coming in at all. The Reiki Professional giving Reiki does not need to instruct the body of the person receiving it in any way. This frees up both the person giving and the person receiving Reiki to relax and enjoy their role in the healing session.

As Reiki is a natural, healing vibration, to the planet and the human body. As such, the human body, generally speaking, will always accept it, unless it has a reason not to. There are reasons other than Reiki that may keep a person from receiving the vibration from another. Reasons for not accepting Reiki can include the person not being able to relax to the point of being willing to accept Reiki from the person offering. This does not always happen for personal reasons, such as dislike or distrust of the person offering Reiki, although in some cases it might. In other instances, the person receiving may not feel comfortable in the room, on the chair, or in the place where the Reiki is being offered. Ultimately, the reason why is less important than acknowledging the fact that there is a level of discomfort present. With that acknowledgement change is possible.

REIKI IS PURE BUT PEOPLE ARE NOT

As discussed in earlier chapters, Reiki is a pure, natural, solid and closed healing system that cannot be altered, manipulated or affected by the Practitioner's energy, state of mind or emotional state. As long as the Practitioner has correctly been attuned and holds their hands in the cupped Reiki position, pure Reiki will come out.

The absence of influence a Practitioner has on Reiki is not true of all energy healing vibrations. Some energy healing vibrations require some form of manipulation or meditative state to provide the healing required to the person in need. Generally speaking, these are subtler energy vibrations that work on different parts to bring about energy healing to the human body as a whole. To that end, a more specialized knowledge of energy, healing and control must be had to use them properly to affect the desired change and healing.

Reiki is different, and its differences have been explained in detail throughout the book. For the purposes of our discussion here, what this means is that Reiki is safe from both the influence of the Practitioner giving Reiki and of the person receiving it. However, it is important to note, that the mind and energy of the person receiving Reiki can be influenced and affected by the mind and energy of the person giving Reiki and vice versa. This has nothing to do with the vibration of Reiki. In fact, the level of influence I describe here is equally true of the person you stand next to at the supermarket, as it is with all the interactions of your daily life; including those with your boss, co-workers and the family members you live with.

Basically, knowingly or unknowingly you can be, and frequently are, affected by the state of mind and emotional state of the people you interact with, as well as people you simply come in contact with, within the world. The person giving you Reiki is no different. I highlight this as a means to explain that if you notice some difficulty or discomfort in receiving Reiki, the problem is not going to be with Reiki, but with the person or an association you may have of the person you are receiving from. To ascribe the problem to Reiki may negatively influence your willingness to use this wonderful healing vibration, when all that is likely needed is to consider changing to a different Reiki Practitioner.

A Special Note to Energy Sensitives

Although the purity of Reiki cannot be altered, manipulated or affected by the state of mind or emotional state of the of the Practitioner, you may find yourself feeling uncomfortable and so unable to receive Reiki from person standing over or beside you. As stated earlier, the reasons for this can be many, but they are not associated with Reiki. I want to emphasize this; the Reiki vibration is as natural to the human energy system as water and air are to the human body, so any discomfort experienced or hesitation felt, is not being caused by Reiki. Instead, what may be happening is that you may be aware from an energetic perspective, not a mental or conscious one, of the quality of cleanliness of the Practitioner's aura, the energetic cleanliness of the room you are in, or of the energetic cleanliness of the treatment table you are asked to lay upon.

These are things that a naturally energy sensitive person, or someone who has become unnaturally energy sensitive from a compromised aura, can be affected by and feel uncomfortable with. If this is the case, whether you consider yourself energy sensitive or not, tell yourself and reconsider having the session because the other great thing about Reiki, which is also what makes it safe, is that you can only receive it from another person if all of you agrees to receiving it.

It is difficult to know in most cases whether you are naturally energy sensitive or if you have been unnaturally made so from a compromised aura, and this is not the book that will go into depth on these things except to say that a good Energy Medicine Practitioner would very likely be able to help you either way.

More Trouble with Receiving

Other reasons you may find it difficult to receive Reiki from another, include but are not limited to: false perceptions and influences that cause you to doubt your personal worth, a practitioner reminding you of a relative, ex-partner or friend, and/or a belief that your need for protection exceeds your need for healing and re-balancing. Of course there are as many individual reasons as there are individuals, and each of these reasons can be remedied if remedy is sought and change desired. While Reiki alone may not be enough to affect permanent change to these problems, it can help. And the start of that help is not necessarily though receiving Reiki from another. Instead, it can start within the safety and generosity of self-care.

THE SAFETY AND GENEROSITY OF SELF-CARE

From the scope of this book, I would say that if receiving Reiki or any healing from another person is difficult or uncomfortable, consider receiving a Reiki attunement yourself and start giving yourself Reiki on a daily and consistent basis.

Your body will never refuse receiving Reiki from you because you cannot reject you, except as part of a mental process that consists of a series of judgments created from societal ideals. Self-depreciation and rejection exist as part of identity, and in most cases created as a means to fit in and be part of a society that is perceived to be able to offer you physical safety and emotional security. So then, rejection of your body, emotions, thoughts, or any other part of you is done through the identity as part of ego. Energetically and biologically speaking, you cannot reject yourself. In fact, your energy and biology will always do everything it can to heal and find balance, regardless of your state of mind or emotional state.

So your body will always agree to accept the self-care provided by giving Reiki to yourself. The challenge may then be what it is for many, which is to remember to give it to you on a consistent basis. "Forgetting" to do it is also part of a mental process and in many, not all cases, a way to deny you the self-care you deserve. Many agree it is easier to place the needs of our friends and family above our own and place us last in terms of providing care and kindness. So for fun then, and as a point of comparison, notice how often you forget to end your day with giving yourself a few minutes of Reiki with how often you forget to brush to teeth.

A Self-Care Case Study

As part of the initiation process in my Reiki Lineage, we complete a 21-day adjustment period following the attunement. During these 21 days the initiate is prohibited from giving Reiki to another. Instead, they are required to give themselves a full session of Reiki each day.

The purpose of this practice is twofold: for students to further embed and fully set the attunement into their energy system, and to spend time getting to know their energy system and the affect Reiki is having on it. This practice will also deepen the instruction provided by the Reiki Master Teacher during the attunement process and it gives students a first hand lesson in the power of self-care.

In my case, I did my practice at the very end of my day, which was before bed each night. I found it so wonderful I've never really stopped. The first thing I noticed was how well and naturally I would fall off to sleep when I was done. Before, my mind would often keep me up either going through the events of my day or setting up the events for my tomorrow.

With Reiki that was gone and I was sleeping better and deeper than ever. I then noticed that I was naturally drinking more water, as if my natural thirst had increased. But what I came to realize was that my thirst didn't increase, the awareness of how much water my body needs in a day heightened, and I naturally responded to the change.

In addition to ending my day with Reiki, I started placing Reiki hands on myself in the grocery store, while I was sitting in a meeting, or on the phone. When I did, I noticed that the things I was engaging in had more life, tasks I was performing became easier and overall I had the sense that I had found what I felt I had been missing to smooth out the edges of life.

I encourage every person on the planet to learn about, become attuned to, and use Reiki as a part of his or her daily self-care practice. I then encourage patience, because while you may experience immediate benefits to using it, it is in the consistent daily use of it that true ease and deep benefits are found. Much in the same way you notice the daily benefit to tooth brushing as fresh breath, but enjoy, with even more satisfaction, the moment you realize you haven't needed a tooth filling in years.

SEVEN

GIVING REIKI

Understanding how to give a full Reiki session that details placement points or positions on the body should come to you as part of the attunement process with a Reiki Master Teacher. Time spent with your Reiki Master Teacher is the student's best resource as the verbal instruction can be accompanied by physical illustrations, and hopefully, the opportunity to practice on another person. For this reason, I will not go into those details and will instead refer questions regarding those to your Reiki Master Teacher. What is discussed here, then, encompasses a broader look at giving Reiki and offers topics for consideration that will further your continuing education on it. For this reason, this chapter is best read after receiving an attunement, as it will add value to the practice of giving Reiki at any level of attunement. If you read this chapter before you have received an attunement expect that it will have less value for you.

To Need Reiki is Human, to Give it is Divine

Once you have been properly attuned to Reiki and have received some basic instruction on how to use it, giving it to another is easy and fun. While for most, giving Reiki may not be as enjoyable as receiving it, it can feel rewarding knowing you are helping another to relax deeply and feel better. In fact, many students and Reiki professionals alike enjoy the natural boost in self-confidence that comes from knowing they can readily provide this kind of healing to others on demand.

In my experience, receiving Reiki can do more for you than helping you relax and feel better. It can also help you to understand yourself and your basic needs in a new way. For while some may perceive this as a spiritual experience, if you look closer, it is more of a deepening in understanding of what is needed for a human being to live an easier, more fulfilling life. To be successful then, requires matching this deepening in understanding with a personal commitment to meet your physical, mental, emotional and energetic needs in equal measure. Without a clear understanding of all parts of us, and here I single out the energetic needs, we are unable to adequately meet them. For often, many supplant an energetic need with a spiritual aspiration, and when they do, they miss the mark on achieving balance in both realms[6]. Receiving Reiki then helps us to meet a need for self-care that in most is being consistently missed. It also enables us to look through a

---

[6] This is not to minimize the need for many to have spiritual aspirations, or the value of them. It is simply to help differentiate between a spiritual and energetic need and help to establish how they relate to one another. For a failure to meet an energetic need will affect spiritual experience by limiting its potential, while meeting our energetic needs can maximize it.

new lens, with which to see and understand the needs of all humans from a micro, or personal, point of view.

Giving Reiki achieves a similar understanding but in a macro sense, which enlarges the lens with which one can see the needs of all humans. This lens provides a less personal point of view, which is equally valuable in gaining such understanding. By giving Reiki to another, you can see how it is affecting change in another. This will give you information about the vibration itself and about overall human health. This level of understanding is exceedingly difficult to obtain from the personal experience of receiving Reiki, even if it is you that is also giving it.

How to Learn Through Practice

The person giving Reiki is a conduit of the natural, human, restorative energy being received. The process of learning through the practice of giving Reiki starts by being an active participant in the process. Many times, I have seen students give Reiki to another imagining they must go into a meditative state or allow a higher power to come in to be truly effective. That, however, is not true of Reiki and is not how Reiki works. And more to the point, being an unconscious, inactive participant will rob you of your opportunity to feel the Reiki flowing through you and feel how the person you are working with is using Reiki to heal and rebalance.

As the person giving Reiki you are the active energy in the room, the person receiving Reiki is the passive. Both the giver and the receiver are having an experience and as such, entitled to get the most out it. The only one that can stop you from enjoying the experience, to the limit of what is possible, is you. It is for this reason that the giver of Reiki can feel assured that there is much to be learned from giving, when a keen, attentive mind, is accompanied by the desire to learn and the personal commitment to stay present throughout the session.

To do this successfully you must avoid mindless distractions to run through your mind, especially lower quality thoughts that contain judgments, either positive or negative, about the person receiving Reiki. I mention this because it is a human quality and one that all humans are prone to.

Also, avoid the temptation to go into a meditative state while giving Reiki. There are certainly some energy healing vibrations that require a meditative state to work, however, Reiki is not one of those vibrations. While a meditative state will not hinder the Reiki vibration, if the person giving Reiki is doing so in a meditative state, he or she will diminish his or her opportunity to fully experience how Reiki is affecting change. An illustrative example follows: While pouring a glass of water does not require a meditative state, neither will being in one, while pouring, hinder the glass from taking water in. However, unless one is extremely well trained in meditation, which most are not, it will likely cause you to overfill the glass or spill over edges, and therefore waste the opportunity of water.

The key to learning more then, is simple enough to explain but truly a challenge to do. First, start by acknowledging that you are a conduit for Reiki to flow through. Second, watch and learn by being attentive of the Reiki and feeling how its being used and affecting the person receiving it. Last, and this is usually the most challenging part, do so while having no (or as little as you can) personal focus on you or on the person receiving Reiki.

GIVING REIKI IN A RUSH

To successfully give anyone Reiki, your cupped Reiki hand is all that is needed. While it is optimal for the person receiving Reiki to be in a comfortable seat or to be lying down, you may not always have that luxury. For example, what if your 6 year old just fell and scraped her knee, or your partner just hit his head on the kitchen cabinet, or your sister is complaining of cramps at the start of her menstrual cycle? In those everyday life instances you're not going to have the time to set up the perfect setting to support a full Reiki session and it would be a waste of time for you to try.

What you can do instead is to respond quickly by offering to place your cupped Reiki hand on the person or near the person (meaning close, but a few inches away from the body). Then simply allow Reiki to do what Reiki does naturally, without any additional intention set, incantation spoken, or any kind of personal interference done on your part. While it may be hard for the ego to accept, but a relief in other ways, you are a conduit of Reiki to come through, so the less of "you" in the way, the more Reiki can be delivered.

WHAT ABOUT SETTING MY INTENTION?

This is an important point, and one that may upset and disappoint some, and provide relief to others. Your intention, regardless of how positive it is, is not necessary for the healing of another using Reiki. In fact, your desire for an outcome can in some ways hinder the person's natural ability to fully receive the pure vibration of Reiki.

How can it hinder? I will explain, but first I'll acknowledge that this is not the popular doctrine given today in regards to healing. But this book is not written to provide you with platitudes or promises of how a life lived in gratitude and good intentions will heal. That is the road, no matter how well intentioned, of the ego, and has no place in Reiki, natural healing, or in understanding Energy Medicine. While it may provide peace to the mental aspects of a person, and in that way make them believe they feel better or are happier, it can become an impediment to true healing.

If you start speaking about things like 'shall this healing be for the greater good' or some version of that, you run the risk of devaluing Reiki. To illustrate this point imagine for a moment how you would feel if your Dentist spoke an incantation like, "Shall the drilling of this bicuspid tooth be for the greater good and bring about good dental health to all sentient beings". It would likely not fill you with confidence that the Dentist feels confident in the quality of her work and is taking full responsibly for her ability to do a good, complete job.

Other effects of uttering an incantation of such is that the person receiving Reiki can knowingly and unknowingly start to feel pressured into feeling better, as to feel better would be the appropriate spiritual response. This can, and often becomes, an impediment to healing as the clients may become insecure, feeling that they have failed if their pain or discomfort is not gone right away. In still other instances, the client can start to feel indebted to the healer. Then in an effort to make the healer feel that her time was not wasted, the client may make up excuses or say he feels better when he doesn't. Worse still, the client may attempt to prop up the healer's ego as a way to shift attention away from him and the healing, and onto the healer. To this I say "Healer Beware", for while it appears to be a tempting nectar to drink, in the long run, you'll choke on it.

Additionally, it is not only the intentions of the healer than can get in the way, but also the false belief that the healer must personally care about the client receiving Reiki to affect change. In this way, a client may try to impress upon the Reiki professional his admiration, or ask questions in such a way to make the professional feel confident that she is the authority in the room. While the motivation to do this is human, it does nothing to further healing, and that is after all, the point.

When instances such as these have occurred with clients in my practice, I remind them honestly that I cannot care about the outcome of their healing. If I did, it will only get in their way. Instead, I offer them my complete attention, focus, the benefit of my training and expertise and then the real and proverbial "I" gets out of their way so that the energy vibrations I use, (in this discussion, Reiki) can work with their innate healing abilities to restore health and balance.

This is what you too can offer: Reiki and the indifference necessary to allow the person receiving it to use it. This is unquestionably easier said than done. This is especially true when you are offering Reiki to someone you care about. So to the parent offering Reiki to a child that just fell and scraped his elbow, remind yourself that you don't worry and hope the Band-Aid will work, you trust the Band-Aid to do its job and then essentially get out of the Band-Aids' way. You can do the same with Reiki.

To the person who is an established Reiki professional or aspiring to be one, it will not always be easy to be indifferent if you have clients that desperately want you to care about them personally, and try to make that so. But it is your profession, and your clients need your expertise and confidence, both of which become compromised if you care about them personally.

HEALING WITH INDIFFERENCE

Healing with indifference is also one of the precepts in the Western medical model. A Medical Doctor, as part of her training, will be indoctrinated in this philosophy as part of her medical education. Medical Doctors, as part of their oath, will heal anyone that needs healing, even if this is a known criminal or an enemy of state at times of war. Equally, Medical Doctors are not permitted to be the attending physician of immediate family members. Both conditions of practice were created to help the profession value humans as a species first, and not to judge or define their value based on affiliations, prejudices or desires for a personal outcome. The desire for a personal outcome, as opposed to a medical outcome, compromises their ability to be truly objective and so leaves them unable to see clearly or understand the full scope of what is required to effectively provide medical treatment to the person in need.

Caring about the general health of a patient and having a strong personal commitment to doing your best work, is different than being personally invested in the health of a singular person in need of healing and in your care. While it goes without saying that Medical Doctors, Energy Medicine Practitioners, Reiki Master Teachers and Healers in all forms of practice and traditions want the people who come to them for healing to feel better, the best ones know that if they make it personal, the care of the person in need will be compromised.

CONSENT FOR REIKI

If you decide to enjoy a Reiki practice that mostly consist of giving yourself daily or consistent Reiki, then the remaining chapter will be of little interest to you. However, if you have any interest in offering Reiki to others as part of providing healing to family and friends, or intend to treat others on a semi or regular basis as a Reiki Professional, then there is an additional skill it will be helpful to develop. That skill will come naturally to some, while others will need to work to develop it. Simply said, it is the ability to feel when a person is receiving Reiki or not.

Generally speaking, most people you will work with will receive Reiki freely and easily. However, it's important to remember that it is the person receiving the Reiki who is in control, and it is they who ultimately, albeit unknowingly, route the Reiki to the area within the body or auric layer that it is needed most. On occasion, you may begin working with someone who you feel and recognize is not taking in Reiki, despite you giving it.

People may not take in Reiki for many reasons and there is no reason to make their reasons personal to you. If you like, you can talk to them about it or not, but whatever you do, do not push Reiki or any type of healing onto to someone who is not ready for it, or is not interested in receiving it. This includes people who say "no", as much as it includes people who say "yes".

So, "no" means no and that is easy enough to understand. Except, some people get so excited about their experience with Reiki, they want to tell everyone about how great Reiki is and want to share that with the world. This can be a good thing to do, but to be effective it must be done with balance. What is increasingly difficult for many to understand, especially about their family, friends and others they care about, is the reality that for some, healing can be more difficult to live with than their existing problems.

So, "yes" can mean no sometimes? Yes, if the "yes" is a purely mental response. In those cases, the "yes" can be misleading and in most cases, the person saying "yes" is not aware that his or her body is saying no. The "yes" can come from people who care about you and genuinely want to support you and your excitement for Reiki. They may even be curious themselves but for reasons unknown, their body at that time says "no". This may change the next time you try, but it is important to always listen to the body, not the words or the sentiment generated by a well-meaning mind. The only way you will know the difference is by feeling if the person you are working with is actually receiving Reiki.

Now remember, Reiki can do no harm, so even if you miss noticing that the person receiving Reiki isn't in fact receiving it, you can rest assured knowing that haven't hurt or caused harm to himm or her in any way. You cannot overdose or have too much Reiki. The body will simply take what it needs and when it is done, will stop receiving. So, if you give too much all that will happen is the person won't receive it and the two of you may have wasted a little time.

UNDERSTANDING THE KICK-BACK RESPONSE

What is also a common occurrence, and another area where your new skill will help, is feeling when the person receiving Reiki is full, or when a particular area of the body where you are providing Reiki is at its limit. This is generally experienced as a sensation I call "kick-back"[7]. And so called because the sensation feels like you have been gently kicked back from the body as it informs the person giving Reiki that it is full. If you are giving Reiki to another and feel kick-back, it is your responsibility to respond by simply moving to another part of the body and start providing it there, as part of the greater sequence of positions you have learned from your Reiki Master Teacher. For example, the right knee area may have its fill of Reiki and the kick-back is simply the body's way of informing you that it is ready to have the Reiki administered on the left side.

In an earlier chapter I mention that the body knows where the Reiki is needed most, and will direct the Reiki there regardless of where the Reiki is being received. This is

---

[7] The feeling of kick-back is similar to the feeling you get when you are pumping gas into your car and the gas tank informs you that it's full. There is a mechanism inside the gas tank of the car that when full informs the outside gas hose to stop pumping gas inside. The human body has a mechanism that feels similar when it has received its full limit of Reiki. This is something to be initially experienced with your Reiki Master Teacher. Please be aware they may use another name to describe this sensation.

true, which on the surface may appear to contradict the last statement made, but with deeper understanding it doesn't. This is because the body is both intelligent and efficient in its use of resources, so when it knows it is receiving a full session or Reiki in surplus, it will take in the Reiki where administered. When receiving smaller portions of Reiki it will route it to where it will be most effective.

CASE STUDY ON KICK-BACK

The first time I experienced kick-back was during my Reiki Level I attunement. My Reiki Master Teacher encouraged me and the other woman I was being attuned with to learn its feel, and so taught us as part of the practice session going over each of the Reiki positions points on the body. Although I picked up and developed the skill pretty quickly, I found my mind wanting to doubt what I was feeling, in an effort to be "sure".

During the practice portion of the attunement instruction, I did not notice a rhyme or reason to the kick-back. As I practiced using Reiki with the woman I had just been attuned with, I noticed that one area would kick-back after only a minute while another part would receive for 3. In time, and after working with many others, a pattern did start to emerge where I noticed that sensitive areas like the heart tend to take in less when compared to other areas such as a knee.

Learning through the experience of kick-back also helped me to find indifference and not take my role in giving a Reiki session personally. It did this by helping me to experience the session as an objective observer acting as a conduit of Reiki.

From that very valuable perspective, I was able to further develop other skills that helped me to see and feel illness and injury, and to understand how Energy Medicine is used as a means to restore health in a greater context. This combined learning helped me to understand clearly, the benefits and the limitations of Reiki as a vibration, and as a practice.

Eight

Limitations in the Practice of Reiki

This chapter has the least information about Reiki as a healing practice or vibration, and the most on some of the pitfalls that can be experienced through its practice. The chapter is written to encourage thought and discussion, and to help explain why and where limitations and misunderstandings can be experienced. Additionally, it is written to show how simple changes in practice and teaching can help you and others reap the benefits a Reiki practice provides.

The topics I go into may create some controversy and disagreement, as I am going against some of the more popular topics/discussions taught and written about Reiki today. I encourage you to read my words without prejudice to know for yourself if what I am sharing here has merit. While it is easier to write something you feel everyone will agree with, it would not be right. What I share here, I share with any and every Reiki student I speak with on the topic of Reiki, and each topic can be used as a point of discussion and exploration for continuing education courses.

DISTANCE REIKI

Distance Reiki is taught as part of a Reiki Level II attunement. Distance Reiki is based on the reality that distance is an illusion. It is a method that was designed for use when there are few or no other options available. Distance Reiki was never intended to supersede or usurp hands-on healing. This is a critical caveat commonly missed when teaching the technique. In the same way that a long distance consultation with a doctor should not take the place of being examined by one in person when that option is available, distance Reiki should not take the place of hands-on Reiki, when a Reiki professional is available.

The reason for this is that while in reality there is no distance; it is almost impossible to ask the modern mind to accept and embody this truth. This is where the effectiveness of distance Reiki starts to decline. There are valid reasons that affect both the person giving the distance Reiki and the person receiving it that make distance Reiki essentially ineffective. This includes the fact that people depend on time as a tenement on which to construct the version of reality with which they understand themselves and the existence of life itself.

In practice, distance Reiki is taught without further instruction on mind or energy control. This further instruction would take considerable amount of time to master and to be honest, generally not within the realm of tutelage most healing professionals have acute interest in. Then again, even if a healer did, the healer, acting as the person giving distance Reiki, is only one part of the equation. In most cases, the person receiving distance Reiki can't help but be aware of the distance between her and the healer giving it.

The awareness of physical distance enables negative thoughts, in the form of doubt, to get in the way of the healing. This often happens even with someone who is asking for distance Reiki and very much wants to receive it. This is because wanting alone is not enough. When it comes to effectively giving or receiving distance Reiki, it is not simply a function of what the person wants, it is also a function of the complexity of the rational mind, and most humans are not taught how to control the mind to the point where desires can counterbalance ongoing mental processes that allow the illusion of control.

It is helpful, then, to understand that without the mind control and energy understanding necessary to be effective from both participants, distance Reiki becomes something more like giving someone a hug and sending well wishes for an easy and speedy recovery. Its intentions are good, and for this reason it is a nice thing to do. However, it is not something that an ailing person should depend upon for healing, especially if the person in need of healing is in need of actual healing.

With that said, distance Reiki can do no harm. In theory distance Reiki works, and on occasion will do what it is designed and intended to do. And for these reasons, distance Reiki is a good and reasonable technique to use and to teach. However, it needs to be noted that distance Reiki was not intended to replace, and so should not attempt to replace, hands-on healing where and when hands-on healing is available. Additionally, if distance Reiki is to be done, it should be done with both participants having realistic expectations of the result, otherwise both participants can begin to doubt the effectiveness of Reiki, not only in distance work, but also in its larger body of practice.

USING REIKI ON ANIMALS

Many books have been written about the benefits of using Reiki on animals. In fact, many offer it as a professional service and/or teach Reiki as a healing system for animals, as well as humans. The problem with that is simply that Reiki is a human healing vibration. It is not an animal healing vibration. Animals, as living creatures, have an aura and a chakra system. However similar, animal energy systems differ from the human energy system and so require different vibrations for healing.

Animals have their own healing vibrations and use them as a way to heal themselves. With that said, Reiki does not harm animals. In fact and in most cases, animals meet Reiki with ease and relaxation, which makes giving Reiki to an animal a fun and enjoyable thing to do. Furthermore, the relaxation Reiki provides can help the animal use their natural healing abilities, with natural animal healing vibrations, to heal themselves. And it is for this reason that Reiki has been misunderstood as a vibration that heals animals. It does not. Reiki will help the animal relax, and in that way will make them feel better, and if that is what you wish to do, then you will do so successfully. If however, your desire is to learn more about how to directly heal animals, Reiki alone will not suffice. To do that and be consistently effective, you will need to learn about and use natural animal healing vibrations.

Reiki and the Pregnant Woman

In some ways it could be argued that no one needs, and can benefit from, Reiki more than a pregnant woman. And while there are numerous ways that Reiki can make the time spent in pregnancy an easier and gentler process, there is something that each Practitioner should be aware of when deciding whether to offer Reiki or a Reiki attunement to a pregnant woman.

A pregnant woman has a double aura. This is because she has her aura and the aura of the developing child. This is the simple energy explanation of why a woman "glows" when she is pregnant. Therefore, her energy system for the time that she is pregnant consists of her energy and that of her unborn child. While the pregnant woman can give consent to receive Reiki, the unborn child cannot. Furthermore, Practitioners and Healers who believe they can ask the unborn child for consent, and get a pure, unbiased answer, generally speaking, cannot. The reasons for this include the person asking not having the energy or mind control to do this effectively; this is true even for those with natural psychic abilities. And to be fair, even if a response was received, the unborn child is made up more of what he or she was before the impending birth, than what he or she will be, once born into the new karma.

Ultimately, what this means is that it is best for the Mother-to-be to receive a Reiki attunement before she becomes pregnant, and then continue to give herself consistent, self-care Reiki treatments throughout her pregnancy and impending recovery, following the birth. The reason for this is not due to a limitation of Reiki, it is a matter of karma. For any person who does not have the energy and mind control required to either get consent from the unborn child, or have the training and ability to separate the energy systems so that healing can be isolated to that of the Mother-to-be, will incur karma with the unborn child. This is not a concern for the Mother-to-be as she already, by virtue of her relationship and acceptance of motherhood, has karma with the child.

It is important to mention here that this is not a mandate of Reiki and in fact, not related to Reiki as much as it is a matter of consent of treatment, and the karma incurred when consent of treatment cannot be given.

BELIEF & LIMITING BELIEFS

For the most part belief is a mental process, which is separate from, but influenced by, experience. Our beliefs are created and used to give us an illusion of control over our lives. That simple truth does not suggest that belief is a negative thing to have, for it is the cornerstone of most people's lives, faith and sense of self. I am simply pointing out the primary function of belief, in an effort to explain how belief or lack thereof, can influence the healing process.

As much as we may want it to be otherwise, for some, it is easier to live with problems, illness, injury and disease than it is to live with healing and good health. There are many reasons for this and absolutely no point in using it as a means or excuse to judge another.

Reiki does not require an individual's belief in it to work. With that said however, if a person doesn't allow or want Reiki to work, it won't. Furthermore, if a person cannot accept the changes that Reiki has made, then that person will engage in activities, mostly unknowingly, that will re-create symptoms that mirror those previously reported. What is key to focus on here is that Reiki cannot be undone once it has affected change, but symptoms can be re-created and over time will be, if Reiki is not used consistently.

Said another way, we humans are a complicated species. On the one hand, we naturally seek meaning to our lives, and belief provides that. On the other hand, we seek distraction, and problems, both real and imagined, providing for us a landscape of distractions to become lost in. One of the many ways we use problems to provide distraction is through self-sabotage, and just one of the ways we do that is to get in the way of our own healing.

If you allow negative thoughts, such as doubt, or are prone to indulge in unresolved feelings of unworthiness, or fear that somehow God would deem such healing as unholy, or the work of lower beings, you will affect what you can receive, and may not benefit from the long term effects Reiki provides with consistent practice. Therefore, the most effective way to experience Reiki is the most direct, by fully experiencing it through the body and its senses. If you are willing to temporarily suspend the need to believe or distract yourself with petty problems, you allow how you feel in your body to inform you of its benefits. What you are looking for is a feeling of general relaxation and a greater sense of well-being that may come in the form of feeling less worry, more optimism, or a simple lessening of general aches and pains.

And don't worry; because experience has always informed belief, so suspending your need to believe temporarily will not change your beliefs. Only experience itself, followed by your acknowledgement and acceptance of an experience had, can change or fortify belief. In some cases, albeit them rare, experience has even been known to release one from the need to believe.

Epilogue

When my daughter was 5 years old she was attuned to Reiki Level I. I agreed to her attunement after her many requests and insistence upon receiving one. While my intention was always to encourage both her and her younger brother Liam to receive one, I was happy the desire and insistence came from her.

Maya was attuned on a Wednesday with two other young girls, one named Giuliana who was 10, and the other named Hannah who was 7. While I was not there, her Reiki Master Teacher told me they had so much fun and I could easily see from Maya's face this was true. But I also saw how much joy her Reiki Master Teacher had with the girls, and how their innocence and wonder made the experience something new for everyone.

Following her Reiki attunement and 21-day adjustment period, Maya has often used her Reiki on herself. In fact, her younger brother Liam will often ask her for Reiki after a taking a fall or bumping his head. What was sad for her however, was when she was told at school after offering it to her friends when they needed it, that Reiki didn't exist; that there was no way that a pure healing vibration that could make them feel better was coming out of her hands. Thankfully, this didn't affect Maya, for she had years of receiving Reiki and knowing for herself what it did for her. It did, however, make her sad that her friends could not feel better right away because they thought she was funny. This is less a story about a little girl, and more one to show how our ideas about what works, and what doesn't, too often get in the way of what is possible.

If only what is seen is real then why are we afraid of the dark? Why do we believe in love? And why do we know gravity to exist? It is because we feel. We feel fear in the dark, we feel the warmth of love in our body and we experience the weight of gravity on our bones, and in so doing accept the invisible adhesive that keeps us on the planet. This too can be experienced with Reiki.

At first instance you may feel heat and after a few minutes relaxed. In time you may start to notice that you feel better, less stressed, more at ease, or an absence of feeling that follows in those that have been battered by stress for an extended period of time. But more than that, with a Reiki attunement and consistent use, you can expect to feel the satisfaction of taking care of yourself and enjoy the boost in self-confidence that comes from knowing that you can and do feel better, and that you are responsible for that sense of well-being.

I have experienced that for myself and I have seen Maya blossom as a result of knowing that she can make herself feel better when she falls and scraps a knee, or after she has had a few too many sweets and her tummy aches, or to just help her fall asleep after a full day.

I have long said, that if I ruled the world (I always say that to the tune of the Nas' hit song featuring Lauryn Hill) that Reiki would be taught in elementary school and that attunements would be given to children as a means to provide self-care and build self-confidence. But I do not rule the world, or govern, or have significant influence over the public school system. What I can do is what so many Reiki Master Teachers do today and what so many, like Mikao Usui and the Masters that followed him, spent their lives doing, which is teaching and attuning people to Reiki and encouraging its use through continuing education and practice. May this book have followed their example and proved itself a worthy addition to the body of knowledge on Reiki. I can say with all sincerity that I am proud of it.

About the Author

Chyna Honey, like most of us, is known to be different things to different people. To some, she is the founder and owner of Café del Soul, two natural and organic cafes located in Marin County, California. To others, she is a Reiki Master Teacher and Energy Medicine Practitioner Teacher, who co-founded Healing for People, which is an Energy Medicine Clinic also located in Marin County. Two young ones call her Mama, one wonderful man calls her wife and many call her friend. What is clear as you cut through the descriptions and titles used to define Chyna, is that she has spent her life helping people by giving them access to better information, offering them better options, and by encouraging the best part of them to emerge unapologetically capable, and with renewed self-confidence. She teaches, mentors and inspires employees and clients alike, and although the scope of each conversation may vary, the central theme found throughout is to help people go beyond the mundane aspects that define their lives so that they may better know and enjoy themselves, and through that understanding, better know and enjoy the world they are a part of.